Plant Ba

Cookbook for Men

Dr. Carlisle's Smash Meal Plan | Quick Recipes for Less Than $10 A Day, Easy to Prepare Even You're Bad in The Kitchen | Build Your Spartan Body in A Stress-Free Way [Grey Edition]

By Taylor Carlisle

ISBN: 978-1-80266-312-9 (Paperback)

ISBN: 978-1-80266-313-6 (Hardcover)

Table of Contents

1. Introduction

This book has been written with the precise purpose of helping, in a healthy and intelligent way, all those men who, for whatever reason, cannot or do not want to eat animal foods, and who wish to approach or undertake a plant-based diet to build their bodies in a natural way, devoting the right time to food preparation without stress and without hating what they eat every day!

Studies show that plant-based food intake can help men in every aspect of their existence, especially

Impotence

The idea that men should eat red meat for better sexual performance couldn't be more wrong. Foods high in saturated fat and cholesterol (meat and dairy products) that clog the arteries that carry blood to and from the heart can also block blood flow to other vital organs!

A diet rich in fruits, vegetables, whole grains, legumes, nuts and seeds protects against clogged arteries, heart disease, stroke and reduces the risk of impotence, which can be an early sign of heart disease.

Prostate Cancer

Prostate cancer is the most common cancer in men. One in eight men will be diagnosed with prostate cancer in their lifetime, and men who eat a lot of red meat or high-fat dairy products are at higher risk. A plant-based, low-fat diet rich in fruits and vegetables, combined with exercise, can help prevent or slow the progression of prostate cancer in men who already have the disease.

Male fitness

Contrary to popular belief, you don't build muscle by eating muscle (meat). Muscles grow with use, and the best diet to fuel them is a well-balanced plant-based diet. The advantage of this diet is that it provides all the good components (complex carbohydrates, antioxidants, and fiber) while avoiding the bad ones (saturated animal fats, animal proteins, and cholesterol; all linked to heart disease, diabetes, obesity, and some cancers). It contains lots of complex carbohydrates: whole wheat bread, whole wheat pasta and brown rice, to provide slow-release energy and fiber to protect heart and gut health. It is rich in antioxidants: vitamins A, C and E, which are especially important for athletes. It also provides a good supply of unmatured essential fatty acids (rich in nuts, seeds, beans, avocados) and plant oils, including omega-3s from flaxseed oil, some nuts and green leafy vegetables, which help keep your heart healthy. It can also satisfy a stronger appetite while providing all the nutrients the body needs to maintain an athletic lifestyle, increase muscle mass and reduce recovery time.

Heart Disease

There are many things men can do to prevent heart disease, including: quitting smoking, exercising regularly and eating a plant-based diet. Avoiding meat and dairy products can help a grown man lose weight, control cholesterol and blood pressure, avoid or manage type 2 diabetes, and ultimately reduce his risk of heart disease.

Ultimately, we all agree that it's not easy to radically change the way you relate to food: it often leads us to euphoria first, but once the excitement has passed, we feel anxious about being changed and wish to return to the previous stage.

The intent of this book is to facilitate the transition to a plant-based diet: gradually and without hating what you eat, you'll get the results you set for yourself sooner than you expect (weight loss, good blood circulation, a more toned and sculpted body, and so on).

Happy reading!

Plant Based Breakfast Recipes

1) *Oatmeal & Peanut Butter Breakfast Bar*

Preparation Time: 10 mitues

Cooking Time: 0 minutes

Servings: 8

Nutrition: Calories 459, Total Fat 8.9g, Saturated Fat 1.8g, Cholesterol 0mg, Sodium 77mg, Total Carbohydrate 98.5g, Dietary Fiber 11.3g, Total Sugars 79.1g, Protein 7.7g, Calcium 51mg, Potassium 926mg

Ingredients:

- 1½ cups date, pit removed
- ½ cup peanut butter
- ½ cup old-fashioned rolled oats

Directions:

- ✓ Grease and line an 8" x 8" baking tin with parchment and pop to one side.
- ✓ Grab your food processor, add the dates and whizz until chopped.
- ✓ Add the peanut butter and the oats and pulse.
- ✓ Scoop into the baking tin then pop into the fridge or freezer until set.
- ✓ Serve and enjoy.

2) *Avocado and 'Sausage' Breakfast Sandwich*

Preparation Time: 15 minutes

Cooking Time: 2 minutes

Servings: 1

Nutrition: Calories 571, Total Fat 42.3g, Saturated Fat 10.1g, Cholesterol 36mg, Sodium 1334mg, Total Carbohydrate 38.6g, Dietary Fiber 6.6g, Total Sugars 3.7g, Protein 14.4g, Calcium 193mg

Ingredients:

- 1 vegan sausage patty
- 1 cup kale, chopped
- 2 teaspoons extra virgin olive oil
- 1 tablespoon pepitas
- Salt and pepper, to taste
- 1 tablespoon vegan mayo
- 1/8 teaspoon chipotle powder
- 1 teaspoon jalapeno chopped
- 1 English muffin, toasted
- ¼ avocado, sliced

Directions:

- ✓ Place a sauté pan over a high heat and add a drop of oil.
- ✓ Add the vegan patty and Cooking Time: for 2 minutes.
- ✓ Flip the patty then add the kale and pepitas.
- ✓ Season well then Cooking Time: for another few minutes until the patty is cooked.
- ✓ Find a small bowl and add the mayo, chipotle powder and the jalapeno. Stir well to combine.
- ✓ Place the muffin onto a flat surface, spread with the spicy may then top with the patty.
- ✓ Add the sliced avocado then serve and enjoy.

3) *Black Bean Breakfast Burritos*

Preparation Time: 30 minutes

Cooking Time: 10 minutes

Servings: 4

Nutrition: Calories 588, Total Fat 17.1g, Saturated Fat 3.4g, Sodium 272mg, Total Carbohydrate 94.8g, Dietary Fiber 16.2g, Total Sugars 5g, Protein 18.1g, Calcium 115mg, Iron 6mg, Potassium 1964mg

Ingredients:

- ¾ cup white rice
- 1 ½ cups water
- ¼ teaspoon sea salt
- ½ lime, juiced
- ¼ cup fresh cilantro, chopped
- 4 small red potatoes, cut into bite-sized pieces
- ½ red onion, sliced into rings
- 1-2 tablespoons olive oil
- Salt & pepper, to taste
- 1 cup cooked black beans
- ¼ teaspoon each ground cumin garlic powder, and chili powder
- Salt & pepper, to taste
- ¼ ripe avocado
- 1 lime, juiced
- 1 cup purple cabbage, thinly sliced
- 1 jalapeno, seeds removed, thinly sliced
- Pinch salt and black pepper
- 2 large vegan flour tortillas white or wheat
- ½ ripe avocado sliced
- ¼ cup salsa and Hot sauce

Directions:

- ✓ Place the rice, water and salt in a pan and bring to the boil.
- ✓ Cover and Cooking Time: on low until fluffy then remove from the heat and pop to one side.
- ✓ Place a skillet over a medium heat, add 1-2 tablespoons olive oil and add the potatoes and onion.
- ✓ Season well then leave to Cooking Time: for 10 minutes, stirring often.
- ✓ Remove from the heat and pop to one side. Take a small pan then add the beans, cumin, garlic and chili. Stir well.
- ✓ Pop over a medium heat and bring to simmer. Reduce the heat to keep warm. Take a small bowl and add the avocado and lime. Mash together.
- ✓ Add the cabbage and jalapeno and stir well. Season then pop to one side.
- ✓ Grab the cooked rice and add the lime juice and cilantro then toss with a fork.
- ✓ Gently warm the tortillas in a microwave for 10-20 seconds then add the fillings. Roll up, serve and enjoy.

4) Cinnamon Rolls with Cashew

Preparation Time: 30 minutes

Cooking Time: 25 minutes

Servings: 12

Nutrition: Calories 226, Total Fat 6.5g, Saturated Fat 3.4g, Cholesterol 0mg, Sodium 113mg, Total Carbohydrate 38g, Dietary Fiber 1.9g, Total Sugars 11.3g, Protein 4.9g, Calcium 34mg, Iron 2mg, Potassium 153mg

Ingredients:

- 3 tablespoons vegan butter
- ¾ cup unsweetened almond milk
- ½ teaspoon salt
- 3 tablespoons caster sugar
- 1 teaspoon vanilla extract
- ½ cup pumpkin puree
- 3 cups all-purpose flour
- 2 ¼ teaspoons dried active yeast
- 3 tablespoons softened vegan butter
- 3 tablespoons brown sugar
- ½ teaspoon cinnamon
- ½ cup cashews, soaked 1 hour in boiling water
- ½ cup icing sugar
- 1 teaspoon vanilla extract
- 2/3 cup almond milk

Directions:

- ✓ Grease a baking sheet and pop to one side.
- ✓ Find a small bowl, add the butter and pop into the microwave to melt.
- ✓ Add the sugar and stir well then set aside to cool.
- ✓ Grab a large bowl and add the flour, salt and yeast. Stir well to mix together.
- ✓ Place the cooled butter into a jug, add the pumpkin puree, vanilla and almond milk. Stir well together.
- ✓ Pour the wet ingredients into the dry and stir well to combine.
- ✓ Tip onto a flat surface and knead for 5 minutes, adding extra flour as needed to avoid sticking.
- ✓ Pop back into the bowl, cover with plastic wrap and pop into the fridge overnight.
- ✓ Next morning, remove the dough from
- ✓ the fridge and punch down with your fingers.
- ✓ Using a rolling pin, roll to form an 18" rectangle then spread with butter.
- ✓ Find a small bowl and add the sugar and cinnamon. Mix well then sprinkle with the butter.
- ✓ Roll the dough into a large sausage then slice into sections.
- ✓ Place onto the greased baking sheet and leave in a dark place to rise for one hour.
- ✓ Preheat the oven to 350°F.
- ✓ Meanwhile, drain the cashews and add them to your blender. Whizz until smooth.
- ✓ Add the sugar and the vanilla then whizz again.
- ✓ Add the almond milk until it reaches your desired consistency.
- ✓ Pop into the oven and bake for 20 minutes until golden.
- ✓ 19. Pour the glaze over the top then serve and enjoy.

5) Sundried Tomato & Asparagus Quiche

Preparation Time: 1 hour 20 minutes

Cooking Time: 1 40 minutes

Servings: 8

Nutrition: Calories 175, Total Fat 5.1g, Saturated Fat 2.3g, Cholesterol 1mg, Sodium 286mg, Total Carbohydrate 24.2g, Dietary Fiber 2.7g, Total Sugars 1.2g, Protein 9.4g, Calcium 118mg, Iron 3mg, Potassium 252mg

Ingredients:

- 1 ½ cup all-purpose flour
- ½ teaspoon salt
- ½ cup vegan butter
- 2-3 tablespoons ice cold water
- 1 tablespoon coconut or vegetable oil
- ¼ cup white onion, minced
- 1 cup fresh asparagus, chopped
- 3 tablespoons dried tomatoes, chopped
- 1 x 14 oz. block medium/firm tofu, drained
- 3 tablespoons nutritional yeast
- 1 tablespoon non-dairy milk
- 1 tablespoon all-purpose flour
- 1 teaspoon dehydrated minced onion
- 2 teaspoons fresh lemon juice
- 1 teaspoon spicy mustard
- ½ teaspoon sea salt
- ½ teaspoon turmeric
- ½ teaspoon liquid smoke
- 3 tablespoons fresh basil, chopped
- 1/3 cup vegan mozzarella cheese
- Salt and pepper, to taste

Directions:

- ✓ Preheat your oven to 350°F and grease 4 x 5" quiche pans and pop to one side.
- ✓ Grab a medium bowl and add the flour and salt. Stir well.
- ✓ Then cut the butter into chunks and add to the flour, rubbing into the flour with your fingers until it resembles breadcrumbs.
- ✓ Add the water and roll together.
- ✓ Roll out and place into the quiche pans.
- ✓ Bake for 10 minutes then remove from the oven and pop to one side.
- ✓ Place a skillet over a medium heat, add the oil and then add the onions.
- ✓ Cooking Time: for five minutes until soft.
- ✓ Throw in the asparagus and tomatoes and Cooking Time: for 5 more minutes. Remove from the heat and pop to one side.
- ✓ Grab your food processor and add the tofu, nutritional yeast, milk, flour, onions, turmeric, liquid smoke, lemon juice and salt.
- ✓ Whizz until smooth and pour into a bowl.
- ✓ Add the asparagus mixture, the basil and the cheese and stir well.
- ✓ Season with salt and pepper.
- ✓ Spoon into the pie crusts and pop back into the oven for 15-20 minutes until set and cooked through.
- ✓ Remove from the oven, leave to cool for 20 minutes then serve and enjoy.

6) Cashew Cheese Spread

Preparation Time: 5 minutes

Cooking Time: 0 minutes

Servings:

Nutrition: Calories 162, Total Fat 12.7g, Saturated Fat 2.5g, Cholesterol 0mg, Sodium 239mg, Total Carbohydrate 9.7g, Dietary Fiber 1.1g, Total Sugars 1.5g, Protein 4.6g, Calcium 15mg, Iron 2mg, Potassium 178mg

Ingredients:

- 1 cup water
- 1 cup raw cashews
- 1 tsp. nutritional yeast
- ½ tsp. salt
- Optional: 1 tsp. garlic powder

Directions:

- ✓ Soak the cashews for 6 hours in water.
- ✓ Drain and transfer the soaked cashews to a food processor.
- ✓ Add 1 cup of water and all the other ingredients and blend.
- ✓ For the best flavor, serve chilled.
- ✓ Enjoy immediately, or store for later.

7) Blueberry French Toast Breakfast Muffins

Preparation Time: 55 minutes

Cooking Time: 25 minutes

Servings: 12

Nutrition: Calories 228, Total Fat 14.4g, Saturated Fat 5.1g, Cholesterol 0mg, Sodium 186mg, Total Carbohydrate 22.9g, Dietary Fiber 4g, Total Sugars 7.8g, Protein 4.3g, Calcium 87mg, Iron 2mg, Potassiuminutes

Ingredients:

- 1 cup unsweetened plant milk
- 1 tablespoon ground flaxseed
- 1 tablespoon almond meal
- 1 tablespoon maple syrup
- 1 teaspoon vanilla extract
- 1 teaspoon cinnamon
- 2 teaspoons nutritional yeast
- ¾ cup frozen blueberries
- 9 slices soft bread
- ¼ cup oats
- 1/3 cup raw pecans
- ¼ cup coconut sugar
- 3 tablespoons coconut butter, at room temperature
- 1/8 teaspoon sea salt
- 9 slices bread, each cut into 4

Directions:

- ✓ Preheat your oven to 375°F and grease a muffin tin. Pop to one side.
- ✓ Find a medium bowl and add the flax, almond meal, nutritional yeast, maple syrup, milk, vanilla and cinnamon.
- ✓ Mix well using a fork then pop into the fridge.
- ✓ Grab your food processor and add the topping ingredients (except the coconut butter
- ✓ Whizz to combine.
- ✓ Add the butter then whizz again.
- ✓ Grab your muffin tin and add a teaspoon of the flax and cinnamon batter to the bottom of each space.
- ✓ Add a square of the bread then top with 5-6 blueberries.
- ✓ Sprinkle with 2 teaspoons of the crumble then top with another piece of bread.
- ✓ Place 5-6 more blueberries over the bread, sprinkle with more of the topping then add the other piece of bread.
- ✓ Add a tablespoon of the flax and cinnamon mixture over the top and add a couple of blueberries on the top.
- ✓ Pop into the oven and Cooking Time: for 25-25 minutes until the top begins to brown.
- ✓ Serve and enjoy.

8) Smoky Sweet Potato Tempeh Scramble

Preparation Time: 17 minutes

Cooking Time:

Servings:

Nutrition: Calories 200, Total Fat 12.3g, Saturated Fat 2.2g, Cholesterol 0mg, Sodium 224mg, Total Carbohydrate 19g, Dietary Fiber 3.7g, Total Sugars 6.5g, Protein 7.5g, Calcium 64mg, Iron 2mg, Potassium 430mg

Ingredients:

- 2 tablespoons olive oil
- 1 small sweet potato, finely diced
- 1 small onion, diced
- 2 garlic cloves, minced
- 8 oz. package tempeh, crumbled
- 1 small red bell pepper, diced
- 1 tablespoon soy sauce
- 1 tablespoon ground cumin
- 1 tablespoon smoked paprika
- 1 tablespoon maple syrup
- Juice of ½ lemon
- 1 avocado, sliced
- 2 scallions, chopped
- 4 tortillas
- 2 tbsp. Hot sauce

Directions:

- ✓ Place a skillet over a medium heat and add the oil.
- ✓ Add the sweet potato and Cooking Time: for five minutes until getting soft.
- ✓ Add the onion and Cooking Time: for another five minutes until soft.
- ✓ Stir through the garlic and Cooking Time: for a minute.
- ✓ Add the tempeh, pepper, soy, cumin, paprika, maple and lemon juice and Cooking Time: for two more minutes.
- ✓ Serve with the optional extras then enjoy.

9) *Fluffy Garbanzo Bean Omelet*

Preparation Time: 20 minutes

Cooking Time: 7 minutes

Servings: 2

Nutrition: Calories 104, Total Fat 1.3g, Saturated Fat 0.2g, Cholesterol 0mg, Sodium 419mg, Total Carbohydrate 17.9g, Dietary Fiber 4.6g, Total Sugars 4.7g, Protein 6.6g, Calcium 69mg, Iron 3mg, Potassium 423mg

Ingredients:

- ¼ cup besan flour
- 1 tablespoon nutritional yeast
- ½ teaspoon baking powder
- ¼ teaspoon turmeric
- ½ teaspoon chopped chives
- ¼ teaspoon garlic powder
- 1/8 teaspoon black pepper
- ½ teaspoon Ener-G egg replacer
- ¼ cup water
- ½ cup Romaine Leafy Green Fresh

Express

- ½ cup Veggies
- 1 tablespoon Salsa
- 1 tablespoon Ketchup
- 1 tablespoon Hot sauce
- 1 tablespoon Parsley

Directions:

- ✓ Grab a medium bowl and combine all the ingredients except the greens and veggies. Leave to stand for five minutes.
- ✓ Place a skillet over a medium heat and add the oil.
- ✓ Pour the batter into the pan, spread and Cooking Time: for 3-5 minutes until the edges pull away from the pan.
- ✓ Add the greens and the veggies of your choice then fold the omelet over.
- ✓ Cooking Time: for 2 more minutes then pop onto a plate.
- ✓ Serve with the topping of your choice.
- ✓ Serve and enjoy.

10) *Easy Hummus Toast*

Preparation Time: 10 minutes

Cooking Time: 0 minutes

Servings:1

Nutrition: Calories 445, Total Fat 16.3g, Saturated Fat 2.2g, Cholesterol 0mg, Sodium 597mg, Total Carbohydrate 54.5g, Dietary Fiber 10.5g, Total Sugars 6.1g, Protein 22.6g, Calcium 116mg, Iron 6mg, Potassium 471mg

Ingredients:

- 2 slices sprouted wheat bread
- ¼ cup hummus
- 1 tablespoon hemp seeds
- 1 tablespoon roasted unsalted sunflower seeds

Directions:

- ✓ Start by toasting your bread.
- ✓ Top with the hummus and seeds then eat!

11) *Chilled Cantaloupe Smoothie*

Preparation Time: 10 minutes

Cooking Time:

Servings:2

Nutrition: Calories 349, Total Fat 13.1g, Saturated Fat 11.3g, Cholesterol 0mg, Sodium 104mg, Total Carbohydrate 50.5g, Dietary Fiber 5.5g, Total Sugars 46.4g, Protein 6.5g, Vitamin D 0mcg, Calcium 117mg, Iron 5mg, Potassium 1320mg

Ingredients:

- 1½ cups cantaloupe, diced
- 2 Tbsp frozen orange juice concentrate
- ¼ cup white wine
- 2 ice cubes
- 1 Tbsp lemon juice
- ½ cup Mint leaves, for garnish

Directions:

- ✓ Blend all ingredients to create a smooth mixture.
- ✓ Top with mint leaves, and serve.

12) Hot Sausage and Pepper Breakfast Casserole

Preparation Time: 57 minutes

Cooking Time: 50 minutes

Servings:8

Nutrition: Calories 263, Total Fat 8.2g, Saturated Fat 1g, Cholesterol 0mg, Sodium 673mg, Total Carbohydrate 31.8g, Dietary Fiber 3.4g, Total Sugars 3.6g, Protein 12.9g, Calcium 239mg, Iron 3mg, Potassium 377mg

Ingredients:

- 10 cup white bread, cubed
- 2¾ cups ice water
- 1 ¼ cup plant-based unsweetened creamer
- 2 tablespoons extra-virgin olive oil
- 3 vegan sausage, sliced
- 1 bell pepper, seeded and chopped
- 1 medium onion, chopped
- 2 garlic cloves, minced
- 5 cups spinach leaves
- 1 cup vegan parmesan, grated
- 1 teaspoon ground sea salt, or to taste
- ½ teaspoon ground nutmeg
- ½ teaspoon ground black pepper
- 1 tablespoon fresh parsley, chopped
- 1 teaspoon fresh rosemary, chopped
- 1 teaspoon fresh thyme, chopped
- 1 teaspoon fresh oregano, chopped
- 1 tablespoon vegan butter

Directions:

- ✓ Preheat your oven to 375°F and grease a 13" x 8" baking dish.
- ✓ Grab a medium bowl and add the water, milk and nutmeg. Whisk well until combined.
- ✓ Pop a skillet over a medium heat and add the oil.
- ✓
- ✓ Add the sausage to the pan and Cooking Time: for 8-10 minutes until browned. Remove from the pan and pop to one side.
- ✓ Add the onions and Cooking Time: for 3 minutes.
- ✓ Add the peppers and Cooking Time: for 5 minutes.
- ✓ Add the garlic, salt and pepper and Cooking Time: for 2 minutes then remove from the pan and pop to one side.
- ✓ Add the spinach to the pan and Cooking Time: until wilted.
- ✓ Remove the spinach from the pan then chop. Squeeze out the water.
- ✓ Grab the greased baking dish and add half the cubed bread to the bottom.
- ✓ Add half the spinach to the top followed by half the spinach and half of the onion and pepper mixture.
- ✓ Sprinkle with half the parmesan then repeat.
- ✓ Whisk the egg mixture again then pour over the casserole.
- ✓ Pop into the oven and bake for 30 minutes until browned.
- ✓ Serve and enjoy.

13) High Protein Peanut Butter Smoothie

Preparation Time: 3 minutes

Cooking Time:

Servings: 2

Nutrition: Calories 687, Total Fat 50.4g, Saturated Fat 38g, Cholesterol 0mg, Sodium 176mg, Total Carbohydrate 46.5g, Dietary Fiber 9.9g, Total Sugars 23.7g, Protein 20.4g, Vitamin D 0mcg, Calcium 150mg, Iron 8mg, Potassium 979mg

Ingredients:

- 2 cups kale
- 1 banana
- 2 tbsp. hemp seeds
- 1 tbsp. peanut butter
- 2/3 cup water
- 2 cups ice
- 1 cup almond or cashew milk
- 2 tbsp. cacao powder
- 1 scoop Vega vanilla protein powder

Directions:

- ✓ Pop the kale and banana in a blender, then add the hemp seeds and peanut butter.
- ✓ Add the milk, water and ice and blend until ingredients are combined.
- ✓ Add the protein powder.
- ✓ Pour into glasses and serve.

14)Pineapple and Kale Smoothie

Preparation Time: 3 minutes

Cooking Time:

Servings: 2

Nutrition: Calories 509, Total Fat 8.9g, Saturated Fat 3.3g, Cholesterol 10mg, Sodium 127mg, Total Carbohydrate 87.1g, Dietary Fiber 10.3g, Total Sugars 55.3g, Protein 30.6g, Vitamin D 0mcg, Calcium 438mg, Iron 5mg, Potassium 1068mg

Ingredients:

- 1 cup Greek yogurt
- 1½ cups cubed pineapple
- 3 cups baby kale
- 1 cucumber
- 2 tbsp, hemp seeds

Directions:

- ✓ Pop everything in a blender and blitz
- ✓ Pour into glasses and serve.

15)Vanilla and Almond Smoothie

Preparation Time: 3 minutes

Cooking Time:

Servings:1

Nutrition: Calories 415, Total Fat 33.8g, Saturated Fat 1.8g, Cholesterol 0mg, Sodium 108mg, Total Carbohydrate 18.2g, Dietary Fiber 7.9g, Total Sugars 2g, Protein 42.1g, Vitamin D 0mcg, Calcium 255mg, Iron 9mg, Potassium 351mg

Ingredients:

- 2 scoops vegan vanilla protein powder
- ½ cup almonds
- 1 cup water

Directions:

- ✓ Pop everything in a blender and blitz
- ✓ Pour into glasses and serve.

16)Berry Blast Smoothie

Preparation Time: 3 minutes

Cooking Time:

Servings: 2

Nutrition: Calories 404, Total Fat 30.4g, Saturated Fat 25.5g, Cholesterol 0mg, Sodium 22mg, Total Carbohydrate 34.5g, Dietary Fiber 12.5g, Total Sugars 19.6g, Protein 6.3g, Vitamin D 0mcg, Calcium 112mg, Iron 4mg, Potassium 581mg

Ingredients:

- 1 cup raspberries
- 1 cup frozen blueberries
- 1 cup frozen blackberries
- 1 cup almond milk
- ¼ cup Soy Yogurt

Directions:

- ✓ Pop everything in a blender and blitz
- ✓ Pour into glasses and serve.

17) Choc-Banana Smoothie

Preparation Time: 3 minutes

Cooking Time:

Servings: 2

Nutrition: Calories 676, Total Fat 52.3g, Saturated Fat 38.1g, Cholesterol 0mg, Sodium 46mg, Total Carbohydrate 41.6g, Dietary Fiber 8.7g, Total Sugars 25.2g, Protein 22.4g, Vitamin D 0mcg, Calcium 80mg, Iron 6mg, Potassium 528mg

Ingredients:

- 1 banana
- 2 tbsp. hemp seeds
- 2/3 cup water
- 2 cups ice
- 1 cup almond or cashew milk
- 2 scoop Vegan chocolate protein powder
- 2 tbsp. cacao powder

Directions:

- ✓ Pop everything in a blender and blitz
- ✓ Pour into glasses and serve.

18) Greens and Berry Smoothie

Preparation Time: 3 minutes

Cooking Time:

Servings: 2

Nutrition: Calories 298, Saturated Fat 19.3g, Cholesterol 0mg, Sodium 29mg, Total Carbohydrate 20g, Dietary Fiber 7.4g, Total Sugars 8g, Protein 4.7g, Vitamin D 0mcg, Calcium 114mg, Iron 3mg, Potassium 520mg

Ingredients:

- 1 cup frozen berries
- 1 cup kale or spinach
- ¾ cup milk almond, oat or coconut milk
- ½ tbsp chia seeds

Directions:

- ✓ Pop everything in a blender and blitz
- ✓ Pour into glasses and serve.

19) Peanut Butter Banana Quinoa Bowl

Preparation Time: 15 minutes

Cooking Time: 15 minutes

Servings:2

Nutrition: Calories 718 Total Fat 29.6g

Total Carbohydrate 90.3g Dietary Fiber 17.5g

Total Sugars 14.5g Protein 30.4g

Ingredients:

- 175ml unsweetened soy milk
- 85g uncooked quinoa
- ½ teaspoon Ceylon cinnamon
- 10g chia seeds
- 30g organic peanut butter
- 30ml unsweetened almond milk
- 10g raw cocoa powder
- 5 drops liquid stevia
- 1 small banana, peeled, sliced

Directions:

- ✓ In a saucepan, bring soy milk, quinoa, and Ceylon cinnamon to a boil.
- ✓ Reduce heat and simmer 15 minutes.
- ✓ Remove from the heat and stir in Chia seeds. Cover the saucepan with lid and place aside for 15 minutes.
- ✓ In the meantime, microwave peanut butter and almond milk for 30 seconds on high. Remove and stir until runny. Repeat the process if needed.
- ✓ Stir in raw cocoa powder and Stevia.
- ✓ To serve; fluff the quinoa with fork and transfer in a bowl.
- ✓ Top with sliced banana.
- ✓ Drizzle the quinoa with peanut butter.
- ✓ Serve.

20) Orange Pumpkin Pancakes

Preparation Time:

Cooking Time:

Servings:

Nutrition: Calories 301 Total Fat 12.6g

Total Carbohydrate 41.7g Dietary Fiber 7.2g

Total Sugars 9.9g Protein 8.1g

Ingredients:

- 10g ground flax meal
- 45ml water
- 235ml unsweetened soy milk
- 15ml lemon juice
- 60g buckwheat flour
- 60g all-purpose flour
- 8g baking powder, aluminum-free
- 2 teaspoons finely grated orange zest
- 25g white chia seeds
- 120g organic pumpkin puree (or just bake the pumpkin and puree the flesh
- 30ml melted and cooled coconut oil
- 5ml vanilla paste
- 30ml pure maple syrup

Directions:

- ✓ Combine ground flax meal with water in a small bowl. Place aside for 10 minutes.
- ✓ Combine almond milk and cider vinegar in a medium bowl. Place aside for 5 minutes.
- ✓ In a separate large bowl, combine buckwheat flour, all-purpose flour, baking powder, orange zest, and chia seeds.
- ✓ Pour in almond milk, along with pumpkin puree, coconut oil, vanilla, and maple syrup.
- ✓ Whisk together until you have a smooth batter.
- ✓ Heat large non-stick skillet over medium- high heat. Brush the skillet gently with some coconut oil.
- ✓ Pour 60ml of batter into skillet. Cooking Time: the pancake for 1 minute, or until bubbles appear on the surface.
- ✓ Lift the pancake gently with a spatula and flip.
- ✓ Cooking Time: 1 ½ minutes more. Slide the pancake onto a plate. Repeat with the remaining batter.
- ✓ Serve warm.

21) Breakfast Oat Brownies

Preparation Time: 10 minutes

Cooking Time: 40 minutes

Servings: 2

Nutrition: Calories 309 Total Fat 15.3g

Total Carbohydrate 32.2g Dietary Fiber 9.2g

Total Sugars 9.1g Protein 13.7g

Ingredients:

- 180g old-fashioned rolled oats
- 80g peanut flour
- 30g chickpea flour
- 25g flax seeds meal
- 5g baking powder, aluminum-free
- ½ teaspoon baking soda
- 5ml vanilla paste
- 460ml unsweetened vanilla soy milk
- 80g organic applesauce
- 55g organic pumpkin puree
- 45g organic peanut butter
- 5ml liquid stevia extract
- 25g slivered almonds

Directions:

- ✓ Preheat oven to 180C/350F.
- ✓ Line 18cm baking pan with parchment paper, leaving overhanging sides.
- ✓ In a large bowl, combine oats, peanut flour, chickpea flour, flax seeds, baking powder, and baking soda.
- ✓ In a separate bowl, whisk together vanilla paste, soy milk, applesauce. Pumpkin puree, peanut butter, and stevia.
- ✓ Fold the liquid ingredients into dry ones and stir until incorporated.
- ✓ Pour the batter into the prepared baking pan.
- ✓ Sprinkle evenly with slivered almonds.
- ✓ Bake the oat brownies for 40 minutes.
- ✓ Remove from the oven and place aside to cool.
- ✓ Slice and serve.

22) Spinach Tofu Scramble With Sour Cream

Preparation Time: 10 minutes

Cooking Time: 15 minutes

Servings:2

Nutrition: Calories 411 Total Fat 26.5g

Total Carbohydrate 23.1g

Dietary Fiber 5.9g Total Sugars 6.3g Protein 25g

Ingredients:

Sour cream:

- 75g raw cashews, soaked overnight
- 30ml lemon juice
- 5g nutritional yeast
- 60ml water
- 1 good pinch salt

Tofu scramble:

- 15ml olive oil
- 1 small onion, diced
- 1 clove garlic, minced
- 400 firm tofu, pressed, crumbled
- ½ teaspoon ground cumin
- ½ teaspoon curry powder
- ½ teaspoon turmeric
- 2 tomatoes, diced
- 30g baby spinach
- Salt, to taste

Directions:

- ✓ Make the cashew sour cream; rinse and drain soaked cashews.
- ✓ Place the cashews, lemon juice, nutritional yeast, water, and salt in a food processor.
- ✓ Blend on high until smooth, for 5-6 minutes.
- ✓ Transfer to a bowl and place aside.
- ✓ Make the tofu scramble; heat olive oil in a skillet.
- ✓ Add onion and Cooking Time: 5 minutes over medium-high.
- ✓ Add garlic, and Cooking Time: stirring, for 1 minute.
- ✓ Add crumbled tofu, and stir to coat with oil.
- ✓ Add the cumin, curry, and turmeric. Cooking Time: the tofu for 2 minutes.
- ✓ Add the tomatoes and Cooking Time: for 2 minutes.
- ✓ Add spinach and cook, tossing until completely wilted, about 1 minute.
- ✓ Transfer tofu scramble on the plate.
- ✓ Top with a sour cream and serve.

23) Overnight Chia Oats

Preparation Time: 15minutes + inactive time

Cooking Time: 20 minutes

Servings: 4

Nutrition: Calories 362 Total Fat 13.4g

Total Carbohydrate 52.6g

Dietary Fiber 17.4g Total Sugars 24.6g Protein 12.4g

Ingredients:

- 470ml full-fat soy milk
- 90g old-fashioned rolled oats
- 40g chia seeds
- 15ml pure maple syrup
- 25g crushed pistachios
- Blackberry Jam:
- 500g blackberries
- 45ml pure maple syrup
- 30ml water
- 45g chia seeds
- 15ml lemon juice

Directions:

- ✓ Make the oats; in a large bowl, combine soy milk, oats, chia seeds, and maple syrup.
- ✓ Cover and refrigerate overnight.
- ✓ Make the jam; combine blackberries, maple syrup, and water in a saucepan.
- ✓ Simmer over medium heat for 10 minutes.
- ✓ Add the chia seeds and simmer the blackberries for 10 minutes.
- ✓ Remove from heat and stir in lemon juice. Mash the blackberries with a fork and place aside to cool.
- ✓ Assemble; divide the oatmeal among four serving bowls.
- ✓ Top with each bowl blackberry jam.
- ✓ Sprinkle with pistachios before serving.

24) Mexican Breakfast

Preparation Time: 10 minutes

Cooking Time: 10 minutes

Servings:4

Nutrition: Calories 476 Total Fat 21.9g

Total Carbohydrate 52.4g Dietary Fiber 19.5g

Total Sugars 5.3g Protein 17.1g

Ingredients:

- 170g cherry tomatoes, halved
- 1 small red onion, chopped
- 25ml lime juice
- 50ml olive oil
- 1 clove garlic, minced
- 1 teaspoon red chili flakes
- 1 teaspoon ground cumin
- 700g can black beans* (or cooked beans), rinsed
- 4 slices whole-grain bread
- 1 avocado, peeled, pitted
- Salt, to taste

Directions:

- ✓ Combine tomatoes, onion, lime juice, and 15ml olive oil in a bowl.
- ✓ Season to taste and place aside.
- ✓ Heat 2 tablespoons olive oil in a skillet.
- ✓ Add onion and Cooking Time: 4 minutes over medium-high heat.
- ✓ Add garlic and Cooking Time: stirring for 1 minute.
- ✓ Add red chili flakes and cumin. Cooking Time: for 30 seconds.
- ✓ Add beans and Cooking Time: tossing gently for 2 minutes.
- ✓ Stir in ¾ of the tomato mixture and season to taste.
- ✓ Remove from heat.
- ✓ Slice the avocado very thinly.
- ✓ Spread the beans mixture over bread slices. Top with remaining tomato and sliced avocado.
- ✓ Serve.

25) Amaranth Quinoa Porridge

Preparation Time: 5 minutes

Cooking Time: 35 minutes

Servings:2

Nutrition: Calories 474 Total Fat 13.3g Total Carbohydrate 73.2g Dietary Fiber 8.9g Total Sugars 10g Protein 17.8g

Ingredients:

- 85g quinoa
- 70g amaranth
- 460ml water
- 115ml unsweetened soy milk
- ½ teaspoon vanilla paste
- 15g almond butter
- 30ml pure maple syrup
- 10g raw pumpkin seeds
- 10g pomegranate seeds

Directions:

- ✓ Combine quinoa, amaranth, and water.
- ✓ Bring to a boil over medium-high heat.
- ✓ Reduce heat and simmer the grains, stirring occasionally, for 20 minutes.
- ✓ Stir in milk and maple syrup.
- ✓ Simmer for 6-7 minutes. Remove from the heat and stir in vanilla, and almond butter.
- ✓ Allow the mixture to stand for 5 minutes.
- ✓ Divide the porridge between two bowls.
- ✓ Top with pumpkin seeds and pomegranate seeds.
- ✓ Serve.

Plant Based Soup & Stew Recipes

26)Herby Cheddar Soup

Preparation Time: 12 minutes

Cooking Time: 23 minutes

Servings: 4

Nutrition: Calories 775, Total Fat 57.42g, Total Carbs 8.63g, Fiber 2.1g, Net Carbs 6.53g, Protein 18.2g

Ingredients:

- 5 tbsp butter
- 6 slices vegan bacon, chopped
- 1 small yellow onion, roughly chopped
- 3 garlic cloves, minced
- 2 tbsp finely chopped rosemary
- 1 tbsp chopped fresh oregano
- 1 tbsp chopped fresh tarragon
- 2 cups peeled and cubed parsnips
- 3 ½ cups vegetable broth
- Salt and freshly ground black pepper to taste
- 1 cup unsweetened almond milk
- 1 cup grated cheddar cheese
- 2 tbsp chopped scallions for garnishing

Directions:

- ✓ Over medium heat, melt 1 tablespoon of butter in a large saucepan. Fry in vegan bacon until browned and crispy, 5 minutes. Transfer to a paper towel-lined plate and set aside.
- ✓ Melt remaining butter in the same pot and sauté onion, garlic, rosemary, oregano, and tarragon until fragrant, 3 minutes.
- ✓ Stir in parsnips and vegetable broth, season with salt and black pepper, and Cooking Time: (covereduntil parsnips soften, 10 to 12 minutes.
- ✓ Using an immersion blender, process ingredients until smooth. Stir in almond milk and cheddar cheese; simmer with frequent stirring until cheese melts, 3 minutes.
- ✓ Divide soups into serving bowls, top with vegan bacon, and garnish with scallions.
- ✓ Serve warm with low carb bread.

27)Creamy Onion Soup

Preparation Time: 15 minutes

Cooking Time: 1 hour 5 minutes

Servings: 4

Nutrition: Calories 340, Total Fat 23.43g, Total Carbs 7.24g, Fiber 1.6g, Net Carbs 5.64g, Protein 15.15g

Ingredients:

- 1 tbsp olive oil
- 2 tbsp butter
- 3 cups thinly sliced white onions
- 2 garlic cloves, pressed
- ½ cup dry white wine
- 2 tsp almond flour
- 3 tbsp freshly chopped rosemary
- Salt and freshly ground black pepper to taste
- 2 cups hot vegetable broth
- 2 cups unsweetened almond milk
- 1 cup grated Pecorino Romano cheese

Directions:

- ✓ Over medium fire, heat olive oil and butter in a large pot. Sauté onions until softened, 10 minutes, stirring regularly to avoid browning. Reduce heat to low and continue cooking for 15 minutes.
- ✓ Add garlic; Cooking Time: further until onions caramelize while still stirring, 10 minutes.
- ✓ Stir in white wine, almond flour, and increase heat. Season with rosemary, salt, and black pepper, and pour in vegetable broth. Cover pot, allow boiling, and then simmer for 30 minutes.
- ✓ Pour in almond milk and half of Pecorino Romano cheese. Stir until cheese melts; adjust taste with salt and black pepper.
- ✓ Spoon soup into serving bowls, top with remaining cheese, and serve warm.

28) Creamy Tofu Mushroom Soup

Preparation Time: 10 minutes

Cooking Time: 14 minutes

Servings: 4

Nutrition: Calories 923, Total Fat 8.59g, Total Carbs 12.23g, Fiber 4.8g, Net Carbs 7.43g, Protein 23.48g

Ingredients:

- 1 tbsp olive oil
- 2/3 cup sliced white button mushrooms
- 1 large white onion, finely chopped
- 1 garlic clove, minced
- 1 tsp ginger puree
- 1 cup vegetable broth
- 2 turnips, peeled and chopped
- Salt and freshly ground black pepper to taste
- 2 (14 ozsilken tofu, drained and rinsed
- 2 cups unsweetened almond milk
- 1 tbsp freshly chopped oregano
- 1 tbsp freshly chopped parsley to garnish
- 1 tbsp chopped walnuts for topping

Directions:

- ✓ Over medium fire, heat olive oil in a large saucepan and Cooking Time: mushrooms until softened, 5 minutes. Remove onto a plate and set aside.
- ✓ Add and sauté onion, garlic, and ginger puree until fragrant and soft.
- ✓ Pour in vegetable broth, turnips, salt, and black pepper. Cooking Time: until turnips soften, 6 minutes.
- ✓ Add silken tofu and using an immersion blender, puree ingredients until very smooth.
- ✓ Stir in mushrooms and simmer until mushrooms heat through, 2 to 3 minutes. Make sure to stir soup frequently to prevent tofu from curdling.
- ✓ Add almond milk and adjust taste with salt and black pepper. Stir in oregano and dish soup.
- ✓ Garnish with parsley and serve with soy chorizo chips.

29) Kale-Ginger Soup With Poached Eggs

Preparation Time: 10 minutes

Cooking Time: 16 minutes

Servings: 4

Nutrition: Calories 463, Total Fat 30.05g, Total Carbs 8.5g, Fiber 2.7g, Net Carbs 5.8g, Protein 23.69g

Ingredients:

- 1 tbsp butter
- ½ tbsp sesame oil + extra for topping
- 1 small onion, finely sliced
- 3 garlic cloves, minced
- 2 tsp ginger paste
- 2 cups chopped baby kale
- 2 cups chopped green beans
- 3 tbsp freshly chopped parsley + extra for garnish
- 4 cups vegetable stock
- Salt and freshly ground black pepper to taste
- 3 cups water
- 4 eggs

Directions:

- ✓ Over medium heat, melt butter and sesame oil in a large pot. Sauté onion and garlic until softened and fragrant, 3 minutes. Stir in ginger and Cooking Time: for 2 minutes.
- ✓ Add kale, allowing wilting, and pour in green beans, parsley, and vegetable stock. Season with salt and black pepper. Cover and allow boiling; reduce heat, and simmer for 7 to 10 minutes.
- ✓ Meanwhile, bring water to simmer in a medium pot over medium heat. Swirl water with a spoon and poach eggs in water one after another, 4 minutes. Remove onto a paper towel-lined plate to drain water.
- ✓ Turn soup's heat off and pour ingredients into a blender. Puree until very smooth and divide into four bowls.
- ✓ Top each with an egg, sesame oil, and parsley.

30) Broccoli And Collard Soup

Preparation Time: 15 minutes

Cooking Time: 18 minutes

Servings: 4

Nutrition: Calories 515, Total Fat 33.89g, Total Carbs 9.1g, Fiber 4.6g, Net Carbs 4.5g, Protein 38.33g

Ingredients:

- 1 tbsp olive oil
- 2 tbsp butter
- 1 medium brown onion, thinly sliced
- 3 garlic cloves, finely sliced
- 1 large head broccoli, cut into florets
- 4 cups vegetable stock
- 2 cups collards
- ¼ cup freshly chopped parsley
- Salt and freshly ground black pepper to taste
- 1 tbsp fresh dill leaves for garnishing
- 1 cup grated Parmesan cheese for topping

Directions:

- ✓ Over medium fire, heat olive oil and butter in a large saucepan and sauté onion and garlic until softened and fragrant, 3 minutes.
- ✓ Stir in broccoli and Cooking Time: until softened, 5 minutes.
- ✓ Add vegetable stock, salt, and black pepper. Cover pot and allow boiling. Reduce heat and simmer until broccoli is very soft, 10 minutes.
- ✓ Open lid and use an immersion blender to puree soup until completely smooth. Stir in collards, parsley, and adjust taste with salt and black pepper.
- ✓ Dish soup, garnish with dill leaves and Parmesan cheese; serve warm.

31) Chilled Lemongrass And Avocado Soup

Preparation Time: 5 minutes

Cooking Time: 5 minutes + 1 hour refrigeration

Servings: 4

Nutrition: Calories 339, Total Fat 33.3g, Total Carbs 6.58g, Fiber 3g, Net Carbs 3.58g, Protein 3.59g

Ingredients:

- 2 stalks lemongrass, chopped
- 2 cups chopped avocado pulp
- 2 cups vegetable broth
- 2 lemons, juiced
- 3 tbsp chopped mint leaves + extra to garnish
- Salt and freshly ground black pepper to taste
- 2 cups heavy cream

Directions:

- ✓ In a large pot, add lemongrass, avocado, and vegetable broth; bring to a slow boil over low heat until lemongrass softens and avocado warms through, 5 minutes.
- ✓ Stir in lemon juice, mint leaves, salt, black pepper, and puree ingredients with an immersion blender.
- ✓ Stir in heavy cream and turn heat off.
- ✓ Dish soup into serving bowls, chill for 1 hour, and garnish with some mint leaves. Serve.

32) Turnip–Tomato Soup

Preparation Time: 15 minutes

Cooking Time: 33 minutes

Servings: 6

Nutrition: Calories 955, Total Fat 86.65g, Total Carbs 10.5g, Fiber 6.5g, Net Carbs 4g, Protein 19.11g

Ingredients:

- 1 tbsp butter
- 1 tbsp olive oil
- 1 large yellow onion, chopped
- 4 garlic cloves, minced
- 6 red bell peppers, deseeded and sliced
- 2 turnips, peeled and chopped
- 3 cups chopped tomatoes
- 4 cups vegetable stock
- Salt and freshly ground black pepper to taste
- 3 cups coconut milk
- 2 cups toasted chopped almonds
- 1 cup grated Parmesan cheese

Directions:

- ✓ Over medium fire, heat butter and olive oil in a medium pot, and sauté onion and garlic until fragrant and soft, 3 minutes.
- ✓ Stir in bell pepper and turnips; Cooking Time: until sweaty, 10 minutes.
- ✓ Mix in tomatoes, vegetable stock, salt, and black pepper. Cover lid and Cooking Time: over low heat for 20 minutes.
- ✓ Turn heat off and using an immersion blender, puree ingredients until smooth. Stir in coconut milk.
- ✓ Pour soup into serving bowls and garnish with almonds and Parmesan cheese.
- ✓ Serve immediately with low carb cheese bread.

33) Spring Vegetable Soup

Preparation Time: 8 minutes

Cooking Time: 12 minutes

Servings: 4

Nutrition: Calories 196, Total Fat 11.9g, Total Carbs 10.02g, Fiber 5.7g, Net Carbs 4.32g

Ingredients:

- 4 cups vegetable stock
- 3 cups green beans, chopped
- 2 cups asparagus, chopped
- 1 cup pearl onions, peeled and halved
- 2 cups seaweed mix (or spinach
- 1 tbsp garlic powder
- Salt and freshly ground white pepper to taste
- 2 cups grated Parmesan cheese, for serving

Directions:

- ✓ In a large pot, add vegetable stock, green beans, asparagus, and pearl onions. Season with garlic powder, salt and white pepper.
- ✓ Cover pot and Cooking Time: over low heat until vegetables soften, 10 minutes.
- ✓ Stir in seaweed mix and adjust taste with salt and white pepper.
- ✓ Dish into serving bowls and top with plenty of Parmesan cheese.
- ✓ Serve with low carb bread.

34) Zucchini-Dill Bowls With Ricotta Cheese

Preparation Time: 10 minutes

Cooking Time: 25 minutes

Servings: 4

Nutrition: Calories 857, Total Fat 36.33g, Total Carbs 12.46g, Fiber 2.4g, Net Carbs 10.06g, Protein 26.13g

Ingredients:

- 4 zucchinis, spiralized and chopped roughly
- Salt and freshly ground black pepper to taste
- ¼ tsp Dijon mustard
- 1 tbsp olive oil
- 1 tbsp freshly squeezed lemon juice
- ½ cup baby spinach
- 1 tbsp freshly chopped tarragon
- 2/3 cup ricotta cheese
- 2 tbsp toasted pine nuts

Directions:

- ✓ Place zucchinis in a medium bowl and season with salt and black pepper.
- ✓ In a small bowl, whisk mustard, olive oil, and lemon juice. Pour mixture over zucchini and toss well.
- ✓ Add spinach, tarragon, ricotta cheese, and pine nuts. Mix with two ladles and serve.

35) Cauliflower Soup

Preparation Time: 10 minutes

Cooking Time: 4 hours 5 minutes

Servings: 04

Nutrition: Calories 119 Total Fat 14 g Saturated Fat 2 g Cholesterol 65 mg Sodium 269 mg Total Carbs 19 g Fiber 4 g Sugar 6 g Protein 5g

Ingredients:

- 2 tablespoons olive oil
- 1½ cups sweet white onion, chopped
- 2 large cloves of garlic, chopped
- 1 head cauliflower, cut into florets
- 1 cup coconut milk
- 1 cup filtered water
- 1 teaspoon vegetable stock paste
- 2 tablespoons nutritional yeast
- Dash of olive oil
- Fresh cracked pepper and Parsley, to serve

Directions:

- ✓ Add olive oil and onion to a slow cooker.
- ✓ Sauté for 5 minutes then add the rest of the ingredients.
- ✓ Put on the slow cooker's lid and Cooking Time: for 4 hours on low heat.
- ✓ Once done, blend the soup with a hand blender.
- ✓ Garnish with parsley, and cracked pepper

36) Greek Lentil Soup

Preparation Time: 10 minutes

Cooking Time: 6 hours 2 minutes

Servings: 04

Nutrition: Calories 231 Total Fat 20.1 g Saturated Fat 2.4 g Cholesterol 110 mg Sodium 941 mg Total Carbs 20.1 g Fiber 0.9 g Sugar 1.4 g Protein 4.6 g

Ingredients:

- Soup:
- 1 cup lentils
- 1 medium sweet onion, chopped
- 2 large carrots, chopped
- 2 sticks of celery, chopped
- 4 cups veggie broth
- Olive oil to sauté
- 4 tablespoons tomato sauce
- 3 cloves garlic
- 3 bay leaves
- Salt, to taste
- Black pepper, to taste
- Dried oregano, to taste
- Toppings:
- Vinegar
- Lemon juice
- Hot sauce

Directions:

- ✓ In a slow cooker, add olive oil and onion.
- ✓ Sauté for 2 minutes then add the rest of the soup ingredients.
- ✓ Put on the slow cooker's lid and Cooking Time: for 6 hours on low heat.
- ✓ Serve warm with the vinegar, lemon juice, and hot sauce.

37) Broccoli White Bean Soup

Preparation Time: 10 minutes

Cooking Time: 4 hrs. 32 minutes

Servings: 04

Nutrition: Calories 361 Total Fat 16.3 g Saturated Fat 4.9 g Cholesterol 114 mg Sodium 515 mg Total Carbs 29.3 g Fiber 0.1 g Sugar 18.2 g Protein 3.3 g

Ingredients:

- 1 large bunch broccoli
- 3 cloves garlic
- 1 medium white potato
- ¼ cup carrot, chopped
- 2 cups almond milk
- 1½ cups white beans, cooked
- 1 white onion, chopped
- ¾ teaspoon black pepper
- ¼ teaspoon salt
- ½ teaspoon smoky paprika
- ⅓ cup nutritional yeast
- 1 bay leaf
- 1 cup cooked pasta

Directions:

- ✓ In a slow cooker, add olive oil and onion.
- ✓ Sauté for 2 minutes then toss in the rest of the ingredients except pasta and beans.
- ✓ Put on the slow cooker's lid and Cooking Time: for 4 hours on low heat.
- ✓ Once done, add pasta and beans to the soup and mix gently.
- ✓ Cover the soup and remove it from the heat then leave it for another 30 minutes.

38) African Lentil Soup

Preparation Time: 10 minutes

Cooking Time: 20 minutes

Servings: 4

Nutrition: Calories 205 Total Fat 22.7 g Saturated Fat 6.1 g Cholesterol 4 mg Sodium 227 mg Total Carbs 26.1 g Fiber 1.4 g Sugar 0.9 g Protein 5.2 g

Ingredients:

- 1 teaspoon oil
- ½ medium onion, chopped
- 2 juicy tomatoes, chopped
- 4 garlic cloves, chopped
- 1-inch piece of ginger, chopped
- 1 tablespoon Sambal Oelek
- 1 tablespoon tomato paste
- 1½ teaspoons ground cumin
- 2 teaspoons ground coriander
- 1 teaspoon Harissa Spice Blend
- ¼ teaspoon black pepper
- ¼ cup nut butter
- 2 tablespoons peanuts
- ½ cup red lentils
- 2½ cups vegetable stock
- ½ cup packed baby spinach

Directions:

- ✓ In a slow cooker, add olive oil and onion.
- ✓ Sauté for 5 minutes then toss in rest of the ingredients except peanuts.
- ✓ Put on the slow cooker's lid and Cooking Time: for 5 hours on low heat.
- ✓ Once done, garnish with peanuts.
- ✓ Serve.

39)Artichoke Bean Soup

Preparation Time: 10 minutes

Cooking Time: 20 minutes

Servings: 04

Nutrition: Calories 201 Total Fat 8.9 g Saturated Fat 4.5 g Cholesterol 57 mg Sodium 340 mg Total Carbs 24.7 g Fiber 1.2 g Sugar 1.3 g Protein 15.3 g

Ingredients:

- 1 (15 ouncecan artichoke hearts
- ½ bunch kale, chopped
- 2 cups vegetable broth
- 1 tablespoon dried basil
- 1 tablespoon dried oregano
- 1 teaspoon salt
- ½ teaspoon red pepper flakes
- Black pepper, to taste
- 2 (14 ouncecans roasted tomatoes, diced
- 1 (15 ouncecan white beans, drained

Directions:

- ✓ Add all ingredients to a saucepan.
- ✓ Put on the saucepan's lid and Cooking Time: for 20 minutes on a simmer.
- ✓ Serve warm.

40)Chinese Rice Soup

Preparation Time: 10 minutes

Cooking Time: 3 hrs.

Servings: 04

Nutrition: Calories 210.6 Total Fat 10.91g Saturated Fat 7.4g Sodium 875 mg Potassium 604 mg Carbohydrates 25.6g Fiber 4.3g Sugar 7.9g Protein 2.1g

Ingredients:

- Congee:
- 1 cup of white rice (uncooked
- 2-inch piece fresh ginger, minced
- 4 cloves garlic, minced
- 10 cups water
- 14 dried shiitake mushrooms
- Toppings:
- Green onions
- Cilantro
- Sesame seeds
- Hot sauce
- Toasted sesame oil
- Soy sauce
- Peanuts
- Chili oil
- Shelled edamame

Directions:

- ✓ Add all the ingredients to a slow cooker.
- ✓ Put on the slow cooker's lid and Cooking Time: for 3 hours on low heat.
- ✓ Once done, garnish with desired toppings.

41)Black-Eyed Pea Soup With Greens

Preparation Time: 10 minutes

Cooking Time: 5 hrs.

Servings: 04

Nutrition: alories 197

Total Fat 4 g Saturated Fat 0.5 g Cholesterol 135 mg

Sodium 790 mg Total Carbs 31 g Fiber 12.2 g

Sugar 2.5 g

Protein 11 g

Ingredients:

- ½ cup black eyed peas
- ½ cup brown lentils
- 1 teaspoon oil
- ½ teaspoon cumin seeds
- ½ cup onions, chopped
- 5 cloves garlic, chopped
- 1-inch piece of ginger chopped
- 1 teaspoon ground coriander
- ½ teaspoon ground cumin
- ½ teaspoon turmeric
- ¼ teaspoon black pepper
- ½ teaspoon cayenne powder
- 2 tomatoes, chopped
- ½ teaspoon lemon juice
- 1 teaspoon salt
- 2 ½ cups water
- ½ cup chopped spinach
- ½ cup small chopped green beans

Directions:

- ✓ Add olive oil and cumin seeds to a slow cooker.
- ✓ Sauté for 1 minute then toss in the rest of the ingredients.
- ✓ Put on the slow cooker's lid and Cooking Time: for 5 hours on low heat.
- ✓ Once done, garnish as desired

42) Beanless Garden Soup

Preparation Time: 10 minutes

Cooking Time: 4 hrs. 5 minutes

Servings: 04

Nutrition: Calories 305 Total Fat 11.8 g Saturated Fat 2.2 g Cholesterol 56 mg Sodium 321 mg Total Carbs 34.6 g Fibers 0.4 g Sugar 2 g Protein 7 g

Ingredients:

- 1 medium onion, diced
- 2 cloves garlic, minced
- 1 green bell pepper, diced
- 1 red bell pepper, diced
- 2 carrots, peeled and diced
- 1 medium zucchini, diced
- 1 small eggplant, diced
- 1 hot banana pepper, seeded and minced
- 1 jalapeño pepper, seeded and minced
- 1 can (28 ouncediced tomatoes
- 3 cups vegetable broth
- 1½ tablespoon chili powder
- 2 teaspoons smoked paprika
- 1 tablespoon cumin
- 2 tablespoons fresh oregano, chopped
- 2 tablespoons fresh cilantro, chopped
- Salt and black pepper to taste
- A few dashes of liquid smoke

Directions:

- ✓ In a slow cooker, add olive oil and onion.
- ✓ Sauté for 5 minutes then toss in the rest of the ingredients.
- ✓ Put on the slow cooker's lid and Cooking Time: for 4 hours on low heat.
- ✓ Once done mix well.
- ✓ Serve warm.

43) Black-Eyed Pea Soup With Olive Pesto

Preparation Time: 10 minutes

Cooking Time: 3 hrs. 5 minutes

Servings: 04

Nutrition: Calories 72 Total Fat 15.4 g

Saturated Fat 4.2 g Cholesterol 168 mg

Sodium 203 mg Total Carbs 28.5 g Sugar 1.1 g

Fiber 4 g

Protein 7.9 g

Ingredients:

- Soup:
- 1 leek, trimmed
- 1 tablespoon olive oil
- 1 clove garlic, chopped
- 1 small carrot, chopped
- 1 stem fresh thyme, chopped
- 1 (15 ouncecan black-eyed peas, drained and rinsed
- 2½ cups vegetable broth
- ½ teaspoon salt
- ¼ teaspoon black pepper
- Pesto:
- 1¼ cups pitted green olives
- ¼ cup parsley leaves
- 1 clove garlic
- 1 teaspoon capers, drained
- 1 tablespoon olive oil

Directions:

- ✓ In a slow cooker, add olive oil, carrot, leek, and garlic.
- ✓ Sauté for 5 minutes then toss in the rest of the soup ingredients.
- ✓ Put on the slow cooker's lid and Cooking Time: for 3 hours on low heat.
- ✓ Meanwhile, blend the pesto ingredients in a blender until smooth.
- ✓ Blend the soup in the slow cooker with a hand mixer.
- ✓ Top with prepared pesto.
- ✓ Serve warm.

44) Spinach Soup With Basil

Preparation Time: 10 minutes

Cooking Time: 5hrs. 5 minute

Servings: 06

Nutrition: Calories 162 Total Fat 4 g Saturated Fat 1.9 g Cholesterol 25 mg Sodium 101 mg Total Carbs 17.8 g Sugar 2.1 g Fiber 6 g Protein 4 g

Ingredients:

- 8 ounces potatoes, diced
- 1 medium onion, chopped
- 1 large clove of garlic, chopped
- 1 teaspoon powdered mustard
- 3 cups water
- ¼ teaspoon salt
- Ground cayenne pepper
- ½ cup packed fresh dill
- 10 ounces frozen spinach

Directions:

- ✓ In a low cooker, add olive oil and onion.
- ✓ Sauté for 5 minutes then toss in rest of the soup ingredients.
- ✓ Put on the slow cooker's lid and Cooking Time: for 5 hours on low heat.
- ✓ Once done, puree the soup with a hand blender.
- ✓ Serve warm.

45) Red Lentil Salsa Soup

Preparation Time: 10 minutes

Cooking Time: 17 minutes

Servings: 06

Nutrition: Calories 119 Total Fat 14 g Saturated Fat 2 g Cholesterol 65 mg Sodium 269 mg Total Carbs 19 g Fiber 4 g Sugar 6 g Protein 5g

Ingredients:

- 1¼ cups red lentils, rinsed
- 4 cups of water
- ½ cup diced red bell pepper
- 1¼ cups red salsa
- 1 tablespoon chili powder
- 1 tablespoon dried oregano
- 1 teaspoon smoked paprika
- ¼ teaspoon black pepper
- ¾ cup frozen sweet corn
- Salt to taste
- 2 tablespoons lime juice

Directions:

- ✓ In a saucepan, add all the ingredients except the corn.
- ✓ Put on saucepan's lid and Cooking Time: for 15 minutes at a simmer.
- ✓ Stir in corn and Cooking Time: for another 2 minutes.
- ✓ Serve.

46) Caldo Verde A La Mushrooms

Preparation Time: 10 minutes

Cooking Time: 5 hrs. 5 minutes

Servings: 08

Nutrition: Calories 231 Total Fat 20.1 g Saturated Fat 2.4 g Cholesterol 110 mg Sodium 941 mg Total Carbs 20.1 g Fiber 0.9 g Sugar 1.4 g Protein 4.6 g

Ingredients:

- ¼ cup olive oil
- 10 ounces button mushrooms, cleaned, and sliced
- 1½ teaspoons smoked paprika
- 1 pinch ground cayenne pepper
- 1 teaspoon salt
- 1 large onion, diced
- 2 cloves garlic, minced
- 2 pounds russet potatoes, peeled and diced
- 7 cups vegetable broth
- 8 ounces kale, sliced
- ½ teaspoon black pepper

Directions:

- ✓ In a pan, heat cooking oil and sauté mushrooms for 12 minutes.
- ✓ Season the mushrooms with salt, cayenne pepper, and paprika.
- ✓ Add olive oil and onion to a slow cooker.
- ✓ Sauté for 5 minutes then toss in rest of the soup ingredients.
- ✓ Put on the slow cooker's lid and Cooking Time: for 5 hours on low heat.
- ✓ Once done, puree the soup with a hand blender.
- ✓ Stir in sautéed mushrooms.
- ✓ Serve.

47) Shiitake Mushroom Split Pea Soup

Preparation Time: 10 minutes

Cooking Time: 6 hours

Servings: 12

Nutrition: Calories 361 Total Fat 16.3 g Saturated Fat 4.9 g Cholesterol 114 mg Sodium 515 mg Total Carbs 29.3 g Fiber 0.1 g Sugar 18.2 g Protein 3.3 g

Ingredients:

- 1 cup dried, green split peas
- 2 cups celery, chopped
- 2 cups sliced carrots
- 1½ cups cauliflower, chopped
- 2 ounces dried shiitake mushrooms, chopped
- 9 ounces frozen artichoke hearts
- 11 cups water
- 1 teaspoon garlic powder
- 1½ teaspoon onion powder
- ½ teaspoon black pepper
- 1 tablespoon parsley
- ½ teaspoon ginger
- ½ teaspoon ground mustard seed
- ½ tablespoon brown rice vinegar

Directions:

- ✓ Add all the ingredients to a slow cooker.
- ✓ Put on the slow cooker's lid and Cooking
- ✓ Time: for 6 hours on low heat.
- ✓ Once done, garnish as desired.
- ✓ Serve warm.

48) Velvety Vegetable Soup

Preparation Time: 10 minutes

Cooking Time: 2hrs 2 minutes

Servings: 4

Nutrition: Calories 205 Total Fat 22.7 g Saturated Fat 6.1 g Cholesterol 4 mg Sodium 227 mg Total Carbs 26.1 g Fiber 1.4 g Sugar 0.9 g Protein 5.2 g

Ingredients:

- ½ sweet onion, chopped
- 4 garlic cloves, chopped
- 1 small head broccoli, chopped
- 2 stalks celery, chopped
- 1 cup green peas
- 3 green onions, chopped
- 2¾ cups vegetable broth
- 4 cups leafy greens
- 1 (15 ouncecan of cannellini beans
- Juice from 1 lemon
- 2 tablespoons fresh dill, chopped
- 5 fresh mint leaves
- 1 teaspoon salt
- ½ cup coconut milk
- Fresh herbs and peas, to garnish

Directions:

1. In a slow cooker, add olive oil and onion.
2. Sauté for 2 minutes then toss in the rest of the soup ingredients.
3. Put on the slow cooker's lid and Cooking
4. Time: for 2 hours on low heat.
5. Once done, blend the soup with a hand blender.
6. Garnish with fresh herbs and peas.
7. Serve warm.

49) Sweet Potato And Peanut Soup

Preparation Time: 10 minutes

Cooking Time: 4 hrs. 5 minutes

Servings: 06

Nutrition: Calories 201 Total Fat 8.9 g Saturated Fat 4.5 g Cholesterol 57 mg Sodium 340 mg Total Carbs 24.7 g Fiber 1.2 g Sugar 1.3 g Protein 15.3 g

Ingredients:

- 1 tablespoon water
- 6 cups sweet potatoes, peeled and chopped
- 2 cups onions, chopped
- 1 cup celery, chopped
- 4 large cloves garlic, chopped
- 1 teaspoon salt
- 2 teaspoons cumin seeds
- 3½ teaspoons ground coriander
- 1 teaspoon paprika
- ½ teaspoon crushed red pepper flakes
- 2 cups vegetable stock
- 3 cups water
- 4 tablespoons fresh ginger, grated
- 2 tablespoons natural peanut butter
- 2 cups cooked chickpeas
- 4 tablespoons lime juice
- Fresh cilantro, chopped
- Chopped peanuts, to garnish

Directions:

1. In a slow cooker, add olive oil and onion.
2. Sauté for 5 minutes then toss in the rest of the soup ingredients except chickpeas.
3. Put on the slow cooker's lid and Cooking Time: for 4 hours on low heat.
4. Once done, blend the soup with a hand blender.
5. Stir in chickpeas and garnish with cilantro and peanuts.
6. Serve warm.

50) 3-Ingredient Carrot And Red Lentil Soup

Preparation Time: 40 minutes

Cooking Time:

Servings: 3

Nutrition: Carbs: 15.3 g Protein: 6.2 g Fats: 0.3 g Calories: 90 Kcal

Ingredients:

- Split red lentils: 1 cup
- Carrots: 1 cup grated
- Water: 6 cups
- Onion: 1 large coarsely chopped
- Fine sea salt: as per your taste

Directions:

1. Take a large saucepan and add water and bring to boil
2. Add the chopped onions, carrots, lentils and salt and bring to boil
3. Lower the heat to medium and Cooking
4. Time: for 20 minutes with partial cover
5. Add the mixture to the high-speed blender to make a puree
6. Whisk in water if desired
7. Add again to the pan and slowly heat on a low flame for 10-15 minutes
8. Add herbs or spices in between to augment the taste

Plant Based Side Recipes

51) Squash & Pomegranate Salad

Preparation Time: 10 minutes

Cooking Time: 0 minutes

Servings: 04

Nutrition: Calories 210.6 Total Fat 10.91 g Saturated Fat 7.4 g Sodium 875 mg Potassium 604 mg Carbohydrates 25.6 g Fiber 4.3 g Sugar 7.9 g Protein 2.1 g

Ingredients:

- Vegetables:
- 5 cups butternut squash, boiled, peeled, and cubed
- 1 tablespoon coconut oil, melted
- 1 tablespoon coconut sugar
- 1 pinch cayenne pepper
- 1 healthy pinch salt
- ½ teaspoon ground cinnamon
- 2 tablespoons maple syrup
- Nuts:
- 1 cup raw pecans
- 2 teaspoons coconut oil
- 1 tablespoon maple syrup
- 1 tablespoon coconut sugar
- 1 pinch cayenne pepper
- 1 pinch salt
- ½ teaspoon ground cinnamon
- Pomegranate Dressing:
- ¼ cup pomegranate molasses
- 2 cups mixed greens
- Juice from ½ a medium lemon
- 2 teaspoons olive oil
- 1 pinch salt
- Black pepper, to taste
- ½ cup pomegranate arils
- ¼ cup red onion, sliced

Directions:

- ✓ In a salad bowl, add butternut cubes and all the salad ingredients.
- ✓ In a separate bowl, toss all the nuts together.
- ✓ Prepare the dressing by mixing all the dressing ingredients in a different bowl.
- ✓ Add nuts and dressing to the squash and mix well.
- ✓ Serve.

52) French Style Potato Salad

Preparation Time: 10 minutes

Cooking Time: 0 minutes

Servings: 04

Nutrition: Calories 197 Total Fat 4 g Saturated Fat 0.5 g Cholesterol 135 mg Sodium 790 mg Total Carbs 31 g Fiber 12.2 g Sugar 2.5 g Protein 11 g

Ingredients:

- Potatoes:
- 2 pounds baby yellow potatoes, boiled, peeled, and diced
- 1 pinch salt and black pepper
- 1 tablespoon apple cider vinegar
- 1 cup green onion, diced
- ¼ cup fresh parsley, chopped
- Dressing:
- 2½ tablespoons brown mustard
- 3 cloves garlic, minced
- ¼ teaspoon salt and black pepper
- 3 tablespoons red wine vinegar
- 1 tablespoon apple cider vinegar
- 3 tablespoons olive oil
- ¼ cup dill, chopped

Directions:

- ✓ Combine all the dressing ingredients in a salad bowl.
- ✓ In a salad bowl, toss in all the vegetables, seasonings, and dressing.
- ✓ Mix them well then refrigerate to chill.
- ✓ Serve.

53) Mango Salad With Peanut Dressing

Preparation Time: 10 minutes

Cooking Time: 0 minutes

Servings: 04

Nutrition: Calories 305 Total Fat 11.8 g Saturated Fat 2.2 g Cholesterol 56 mg Sodium 321 mg Total Carbs 34.6 g Fibers 0.4 g Sugar 2 g Protein 7 g

Ingredients:

- Salad:
- 1 head butter lettuce, washed and chopped
- 1½ cups carrot, shredded
- 1¼ cups red cabbage, shredded
- 1 large ripe mango, cubed
- ½ cup fresh cilantro, chopped
- Dressing:
- ⅓ cup creamy peanut butter
- 2½ tablespoons lime juice
- 1½ tablespoons maple syrup
- 2 teaspoon chili garlic sauce
-
- 3 tablespoons coconut aminos

Directions:

- ✓ Combine all the dressing ingredients in a small bowl.
- ✓ In a salad bowl, toss in all the vegetables, seasonings, and dressing.
- ✓ Mix them well then refrigerate to chill.
- ✓ Serve.

54) Loaded Kale Salad

Preparation Time: 10 minutes

Cooking Time: 0 minutes

Servings: 04

Nutrition: Calories 72 Total Fat 15.4 g Saturated Fat 4.2 g Cholesterol 168 mg Sodium 203 mg Total Carbs 28.5 g Sugar 1.1 g Fiber 4 g Protein 7.9 g

Ingredients:

- Quinoa:
- ¾ cups quinoa, cooked and drained
- Vegetables:
- 4 large carrots, halved and chopped
- 1 whole beet, sliced
- 2 tablespoons water
- 1 pinch salt
- ½ teaspoon curry powder
- 8 cups kale, chopped
- ½ cups cherry tomatoes, chopped
- 1 ripe avocado, cubed
- ¼ cup hemp seeds
- ½ cup sprouts
- Dressing:
- ⅓ cup tahini
- 3 tablespoons lemon juice
- 1-2 tablespoons maple syrup
- 1 pinch salt
- ¼ cup water

Directions:

- ✓ Combine all the dressing ingredients in a small bowl.
- ✓ In a salad bowl, toss in all the vegetables, quinoa, and dressing.
- ✓ Mix them well then refrigerate to chill.
- ✓ Serve.

55) Cherry Tomato Salad With Soy Chorizo

Preparation Time: 5 minutes

Cooking Time: 5 minutes

Servings: 4

Nutrition: Calories 138, Total Fat 8.95g, Total Carbs 5.63g, Fiber 0.4g, Net Carbs 5.23g, Protein 7.12g

Ingredients:

- 2 ½ tbsp olive oil
- 4 soy chorizo, chopped
- 2 tsp red wine vinegar
- 1 small red onion, finely chopped
- 2 ½ cups cherry tomatoes, halved
- 2 tbsp chopped cilantro
- Salt and freshly ground black pepper to taste
- 3 tbsp sliced black olives to garnish

Directions:

- ✓ Over medium fire, heat half tablespoon of olive oil in a skillet and fry soy chorizo until golden. Turn heat off.
- ✓ In a salad bowl, whisk remaining olive oil and vinegar. Add onion, cilantro, tomatoes, and soy chorizo. Mix with dressing and season with salt and black pepper.
- ✓ Garnish with olives and serve.

56) Cauliflower & Lentil Salad

Preparation Time: 10 minutes

Cooking Time: 25 minutes

Servings: 04

Nutrition: Calories 212 Total Fat 7 g Saturated Fat 1.3 g Cholesterol 25 mg Sodium 101 mg Total Carbs 32.5 g Sugar 5.7 g Fiber 6 g Protein 4 g

Ingredients:

- Cauliflower:
- 1 head cauliflower, florets
- 1½ tablespoons melted coconut oil
- 1½ tablespoons curry powder
- ¼ teaspoon salt
- Salad:
- 5 cups mixed greens
- 1 cup cooked lentils
- 1 cup red or green grapes, halved
- Fresh cilantro
- Tahini Dressing:
- 4½ tablespoons green curry paste
- 2 tablespoons tahini
- 2 tablespoons lemon juice
- 1 tablespoon maple syrup
- 1 pinch salt
- 1 pinch black pepper
- Water to thin

Directions:

- ✓ Preheat your oven to 400 degrees F.
- ✓ On a greased baking sheet, toss cauliflower with salt, curry powder, and oil.
- ✓ Bake the cauliflower for 25 minutes in the oven.
- ✓ Combine all the dressing ingredients in a small bowl.
- ✓ In a salad bowl, toss in all the vegetables, roasted cauliflower, and dressing.
- ✓ Mix them well then refrigerate to chill.
- ✓ Serve.

57) Sweet Potato & Avocado Salad

Preparation Time: 10 minutes

Cooking Time: 10 minutes

Servings: 50

Nutrition: Calories 119 Total Fat 14 g Saturated Fat 2 g Cholesterol 65 mg Sodium 269 mg Total Carbs 19 g Fiber 4 g Sugar 6 g Protein 5g

Ingredients:

- Sweet potato:
-
- 1 large organic sweet potato, cubed
- 1 tablespoon avocado or coconut oil
- 1 pinch salt
- Dressing:
- ¼ cup tahini
- 2 tablespoons lemon juice
- 1 tablespoon maple syrup
- 1 pinch salt
- Water
- Salad:
- 5 cups greens of choice
- 1 medium ripe avocado, chopped
- 2 tablespoons hemp seeds

Directions:

- ✓ Preheat your oven to 375 degrees.
- ✓ On a greased baking sheet, toss sweet potato with salt and oil.
- ✓ Bake the potatoes for 20 minutes in the oven, toss halfway through.
- ✓ Combine all the dressing ingredients in a small bowl.
- ✓ In a salad bowl, toss in all the vegetables, roasted potato, and dressing.
- ✓ Mix them well then refrigerate to chill.
- ✓ Serve.

58) Avocado Kale Salad

Preparation Time: 10 minutes

Cooking Time: 0 minutes

Servings: 04

Nutrition: Calories 201 Total Fat 8.9 g Saturated Fat 4.5 g Cholesterol 57 mg Sodium 340 mg Total Carbs 24.7 g Fiber 1.2 g Sugar 1.3 g Protein 15.3 g

Ingredients:

- Dressing:
- ⅓ cup tahini
- 2 teaspoons garlic, chopped
- 1 medium lemon juiced
- 1½ tablespoons maple syrup
- Salad:
- 1 large bundle kale, chopped
- 1 tablespoon grapeseed oil
- 1 tablespoon lemon juice
- 1 medium beet

Directions:

- ✓ Combine all the dressing ingredients in a small bowl.
- ✓ In a salad bowl, toss in all the salad ingredients and dressing.
- ✓ Mix them well then refrigerate to chill.
- ✓ Serve.

59) Broccoli Sweet Potato Chickpea Salad

Preparation Time: 10 minutes

Cooking Time: 22 minutes

Servings: 06

Nutrition: Calories 231 Total Fat 20.1 g Saturated Fat 2.4 g Cholesterol 110 mg Sodium 941 mg Total Carbs 20.1 g Fiber 0.9 g Sugar 1.4 g Protein 4.6 g

Ingredients:

- Vegetables:
- 1 large sweet potato, peeled and diced
- 1 head broccoli
- 2 tablespoons olive or grapeseed oil
- 1 pinch each salt and black pepper
- 1 teaspoon dried dill
- 1 medium red bell pepper
- Chickpeas:
- 1 (15 ouncecan chickpeas, drained
- 1 tablespoon olive or grapeseed oil
- 1 tablespoon tandoori masala spice
- 1 pinch salt
- 1 teaspoon coconut sugar
- 1 pinch cayenne pepper
- Garlic dill sauce:
- ⅓ cup hummus
- 3 large cloves garlic, minced
- 1 teaspoon dried dill
- 2 tablespoons lemon juice
- Water

Directions:

- ✓ Preheat your oven to 400 degrees F.
- ✓ In a greased baking sheet, toss sweet potato with salt and oil.
- ✓ Bake the sweet potatoes for 15 minutes in the oven.
- ✓ Toss all chickpea ingredients and spread in a tray.
- ✓ Bake them for 7 minutes in the oven.
- ✓ Combine all the sauce ingredients in a small bowl.
- ✓ In a salad bowl, toss in all the vegetables, roasted potato, chickpeas, and sauce.
- ✓ Mix them well then refrigerate to chill.
- ✓ Serve.

60) Penne Pasta Salad

Preparation Time: 30 minutes

Cooking Time: 0 minutes

Servings: 04

Nutrition: Calories 361 Total Fat 16.3 g Saturated Fat 4.9 g Cholesterol 114 mg Sodium 515 mg Total Carbs 29.3 g Fiber 0.1 g Sugar 18.2 g Protein 3.3 g

Ingredients:

- Salad:
- 2 cups roasted tomatoes
- 12 ounces penne pasta
- Pesto:
- 2 cups fresh basil
- 4 cloves garlic, minced
- ¼ cup toasted pine nuts
- 1 medium lemon, juice
- ¼ cup vegan cheese, shredded
- 1 pinch salt
- ¼ cup olive oil

Directions:

- ✓ In a blender, add all the pesto ingredients.
- ✓ Blend them well until it is lump free.
- ✓ In a salad bowl toss in pasta, roasted tomatoes, and pesto.
- ✓ Mix them well then refrigerate to chill.
- ✓ Serve.

61) Sesame Seed Simple Mix

Preparation Time: 5minutes

Cooking Time:

Servings: 2

Nutrition: Carbs: 44.5g Protein: 11.5g Fats: 11.4g Calories: 306Kcal

Ingredients:

- Frozen peas: 1 cup can washed and drained
- Corn kernel: 2 cups can
- Salt: as per your taste
- Sesame seeds: 2 tbsp
- Pepper: as per your taste
- Cashew cream: ½ cup

Directions:

- ✓ Combine all the ingredients
- ✓ Serve as the side dish

62)Roasted Fennel Salad

Preparation Time: 10 minutes

Cooking Time: 20 minutes

Servings: 4

Nutrition: Calories 205 Total Fat 22.7 g Saturated Fat 6.1 g Cholesterol 4 mg Sodium 227 mg Total Carbs 26.1 g Fiber 1.4 g Sugar 0.9 g Protein 5.2 g

Ingredients:

- Fennel:
- 1 bulb fennel fronds, sliced
- 1 tablespoon curry powder
- 1 tablespoon avocado oil
- 1 pinch salt
- Salad:
- 5 cups salad greens
- 1 red bell pepper, sliced
- Dressing:
- ¼ cup tahini
- 1½ tablespoons lemon juice
- 1½ teaspoons apple cider vinegar
- 1 tablespoon freshly minced rosemary
- 3 cloves garlic, minced
- 1½ tablespoons coconut aminos
- 5 tablespoons water to thin
- 1 pinch salt

Directions:

- ✓ Preheat your oven at 375 degrees F.
- ✓ On a greased baking sheet, toss fennel with salt, curry powder, and oil.
- ✓ Bake the curried fennel for 20 minutes in the oven.
- ✓ Combine all the dressing ingredients in a small bowl.
- ✓ In a salad bowl, toss in all the vegetables, roasted fennel, and dressing.
- ✓ Mix them well then refrigerate to chill.
- ✓ Serve.

63)Kale Salad With Tahini Dressing

Preparation Time: 10 minutes

Cooking Time: 20 minutes

Servings: 04

Nutrition: Calories 201 Total Fat 8.9 g Saturated Fat 4.5 g Cholesterol 57 mg Sodium 340 mg Total Carbs 24.7 g Fiber 1.2 g Sugar 1.3 g Protein 15.3 g

Ingredients:

- Roasted vegetables:
- 1 medium zucchini, chopped
- 1 medium sweet potato, chopped
- 1 cup red cabbage, chopped
- 1 tablespoon melted coconut oil
- 1 pinch salt
- ½ teaspoon curry powder
- Dressing:
- ⅓ cup tahini
- ½ teaspoon garlic powder
- 1 tablespoon coconut aminos
- 1 pinch salt
- 1 large clove garlic, minced
- ¼ cup water
- Salad:
- 6 cups mixed greens
- 4 small radishes, sliced
- 3 tablespoons hemp seeds
- 2 tablespoons lemon juice
- ½ ripe avocado, to garnish
-
- 2 tablespoons vegan feta cheese, crumbled
- Pomegranate seeds, to garnish
- Pecans, to garnish

Directions:

- ✓ Preheat your oven at 375 degrees F.
- ✓ On a greased baking sheet, toss zucchini, sweet potato, and red cabbage with salt, curry powder, and oil.
- ✓ Bake the zucchini cabbage mixture for 20 minutes in the oven.
- ✓ Combine all the dressing ingredients in a small bowl.
- ✓ In a salad bowl, toss in all the vegetables, roasted vegetables, and dressing.
- ✓ Mix them well then refrigerate to chill.
- ✓ Garnish with feta cheese, pecans, pomegranate seeds and avocado.
- ✓ Serve.

64) Roasted Squash Salad

Preparation Time: 10 minutes

Cooking Time: 20 minutes

Servings: 04

Nutrition: Calories 119 Total Fat 14 g Saturated Fat 2 g Cholesterol 65 mg Sodium 269 mg Total Carbs 19 g Fiber 4 g Sugar 6 g Protein 5g

Ingredients:

- Squash:
- 1 medium acorn squash, peeled and cubed
- 1 tablespoon avocado oil
- 1 pinch each salt and black pepper
- Dressing:
- 1 cup balsamic vinegar
- Salad:
- ¼ cup macadamia nut cheese
- 2 tablespoons roasted pumpkin seeds
- 5 cups arugula
- 2 tablespoons dried currants

Directions:

- ✓ Preheat your oven to 425 degrees F.
- ✓ On a greased baking sheet, toss squash with salt, black pepper, and oil.
- ✓ Bake the seasoned squash for 20 minutes in the oven.
- ✓ Combine all the dressing ingredients in a small bowl.
- ✓ In a salad bowl, toss in the squash, salad ingredients, and dressing.
- ✓ Mix them well then refrigerate to chill.
- ✓ Serve.

65) Vegetable Salad With Chimichurri

Preparation Time: 10 minutes

Cooking Time: 25 minutes

Servings: 04

Nutrition: Calories 231 Total Fat 20.1 g Saturated Fat 2.4 g Cholesterol 110 mg Sodium 941 mg Total Carbs 20.1 g Fiber 0.9 g Sugar 1.4 g Protein 4.6 g

Ingredients:

- Roasted vegetables:
- 1 large sweet potato (chopped
- 6 red potatoes, quartered
- 2 whole carrots, chopped
- 2 tablespoons melted coconut oil
- 2 teaspoons curry powder
- ½ teaspoon salt
- 1 cup chopped broccolini
- 2 cups red cabbage, chopped
- 1 medium red bell pepper, sliced
- Chimichurri:
- 5 cloves garlic, chopped
- 1 medium serrano pepper
- 1 cup packed cilantro
- 1 cup parsley
- 3 tablespoons ripe avocado
- ¼ teaspoon salt
- 3 tablespoons lime juice
- 1 tablespoon maple syrup
- Water to thin
- Salad:
- 4 cups hearty greens
- 1 medium ripe avocado, chopped
- 3 tablespoons hemp seeds
- Fresh herbs
- 5 medium radishes, sliced
- ¼ cup macadamia nut cheese

Directions:

- ✓ Preheat your oven to 400 degrees F.
- ✓ In a suitable bowl, toss all the vegetables for roasting with salt, curry powder and oil.
- ✓ Divide these vegetables into two roasting pans.
- ✓ Bake the vegetables for 25 minutes in the oven.
- ✓ Meanwhile, in a blender, blend all chimichurri sauce ingredients until smooth.
- ✓ In a salad bowl, toss in all the roasted vegetables, chimichurri sauce and salad ingredients.
- ✓ Mix them well then refrigerate to chill.
- ✓ Serve.

66) Thai Salad With Tempeh

Preparation Time: 10 minutes

Cooking Time: 0 minutes

Servings: 04

Nutrition: Calories 361 Total Fat 16.3 g Saturated Fat 4.9 g Cholesterol 114 mg Sodium 515 mg Total Carbs 29.3 g Fiber 0.1 g Sugar 18.2 g Protein 3.3 g

Ingredients:

- Salad:
- 6 ounces vermicelli noodles, boiled
- 2 medium whole carrots, ribboned
- 2 stalks green onions, chopped
- ¼ cup cilantro, chopped
- 2 tablespoons mint, chopped
- 1 cup packed spinach, chopped
- 1 cup red cabbage, sliced
- 1 medium red bell pepper, sliced
- Dressing:
- ⅓ cup creamy peanut butter
- 3 tablespoons tamari
- 3 tablespoons maple syrup
- 1 teaspoon chili garlic sauce
- 1 medium lime, juiced
- ¼ cup water

Directions:

- ✓ Combine all the dressing ingredients in a small bowl.
- ✓ In a salad bowl, toss in the noodles, salad, and dressing.
- ✓ Mix them well then refrigerate to chill.
- ✓ Serve.

67) Niçoise Salad

Preparation Time: 10 minutes

Cooking Time: 15 minutes

Servings: 04

Nutrition: Calories 205 Total Fat 22.7 g Saturated Fat 6.1 g Cholesterol 4 mg Sodium 227 mg Total Carbs 26.1 g Fiber 1.4 g Sugar 0.9 g Protein 5.2 g

Ingredients:

- Salad:
- 6 small red potatoes, peeled, boiled, and diced
- 1 cup green beans, chopped
- 1 head lettuce, chopped
- ½ cup pitted kalamata olives
- ½ cup tomato, sliced
- ½medium red beet
- Chickpeas:
- 1 (15 ouncecan chickpeas
- 1 teaspoon Dijon mustard
- 1 teaspoon maple syrup
- 1 teaspoon dried dill
- 1 pinch salt
- 1 tablespoon roasted sunflower seeds
- Dressing:
- 3 tablespoons minced shallot
- 1 heaping teaspoon Dijon mustard
- 1 teaspoon fresh thyme, chopped
- ⅓ cup red wine vinegar
- ¼ teaspoon salt and black pepper
- ¼ cup olive oil

Directions:

- ✓ Preheat your oven to 400 degrees F.
- ✓ In a greased baking sheet, toss chickpeas with salt and all the chickpea ingredients.
- ✓ Bake the chickpeas for 15 minutes in the oven.
- ✓ Combine all the dressing ingredients in a small bowl.
- ✓ In a salad bowl, toss in all the vegetables, roasted chickpeas, and dressing.
- ✓ Mix them well then refrigerate to chill.
- ✓ Serve.

68) Spicy Avocado Bites

Preparation Time: 25 minutes

Cooking Time:

Servings: 4

Nutrition: Carbs: 5 g Protein: 1 g Fats: 10 g Calories: 110 Kcal

Ingredients:

- Avocado mashed:1
- Cucumbers:2cut into thick slices
- Lemon: 1 tsp
- Salt and pepper: as per your taste
- Vegan chipotle mayo:2 tbsp
- Spicy roasted chickpeas:½ pack
- Fresh herbs:3 tbsp

Directions:

- ✓ Add lemon and seasoning to the mashed avocado
- ✓ Place on each cucumber slice and press using chickpeas
- ✓ Top with herbs and mayo and serve

69) Roasted Bell Pepper Salad With Olives

Preparation Time: 10 minutes

Cooking Time: 20 minutes

Servings: 4

Nutrition: Calories 163, Total Fat 13.3g, Total Carbs 6.53g, Fiber 2.2g, Net Carbs 4.33g, Protein 3.37g

Ingredients:

- 8 large red bell peppers, deseeded and cut in wedges
- ½ tsp erythritol
- 2 ½ tbsp olive oil
- 1/3 cup arugula
- 1 tbsp mint leaves
- 1/3 cup pitted Kalamata olives
- 3 tbsp chopped almonds
- ½ tbsp balsamic vinegar
-
- Crumbled feta cheese for topping
- Toasted pine nuts for topping

Directions:

- ✓ Preheat oven to 400o F.
- ✓ Pour bell peppers on a roasting pan; season with erythritol and drizzle with half of olive oil. Roast in oven until slightly charred, 20 minutes. Remove from oven and set aside.
- ✓ Arrange arugula in a salad bowl, scatter bell peppers on top, mint leaves, olives, almonds, and drizzle with balsamic vinegar and remaining olive oil. Season with salt and black pepper.
- ✓ Toss; top with feta cheese and pine nuts and serve.

70) Tofu-Dulse-Walnut Salad

Preparation Time: 10 minutes

Cooking Time: 15 minutes

Servings: 4

Nutrition: Calories 237, Total Fat 19.57g, Total Carbs 5.9g, Fiber 2.1g, Net Carbs 3.89, Protein 12.75g

Ingredients:

- 1 (7 ozblock extra firm tofu
- 2 tbsp olive oil
- 2 tbsp butter
- 1 cup asparagus, trimmed and halved
- 1 cup green beans, trimmed
- 2 tbsp chopped dulse
- Salt and freshly ground black pepper to taste
- ½ lemon, juiced
- 4 tbsp chopped walnuts

Directions:

- ✓ Place tofu in between two paper towels and allow soaking for 5 minutes. After, remove towels and chop into small cubes.
- ✓ Heat olive oil in a skillet and fry tofu until golden, 10 minutes. Remove onto a paper towel-lined plate and set aside.
- ✓ Melt butter in skillet and sauté asparagus
- ✓ and green beans until softened, 5 minutes. Add dulse, season with salt and black pepper, and Cooking Time: until softened. Mix in tofu and stir-fry for 5 minutes.
- ✓ Plate, drizzle with lemon juice, and scatter walnuts on top.
- ✓ Serve warm.

71) Almond-Goji Berry Cauliflower Salad

Preparation Time: 10 minutes

Cooking Time: 2 minutes

Servings: 4

Nutrition: Calories 203, Total Fat 15.28g, Total Carbs 9.64g, Fiber 3.2g, Net Carbs 6.44g, Protein 6.67g, Protein 2.54g

Ingredients:

- 1 small head cauliflower, cut into florets
- 8 sun-dried tomatoes in olive oil, drained
- 12 pitted green olives, roughly chopped
- 1 lemon, zested and juiced
- 3 tbsp chopped green onions
- A handful chopped almonds
- ¼ cup goji berries
- 1 tbsp sesame oil
- ½ cup watercress
- 3 tbsp chopped parsley
- Salt and freshly ground black pepper to taste
- Lemon wedges to garnish

Directions:

- ✓ Pour cauliflower into a large safe-microwave bowl, sprinkle with some water, and steam in microwave for 1 to 2 minutes or until softened.
- ✓ In a large salad bowl, combine cauliflower, tomatoes, olives, lemon zest and juice, green onions, almonds, goji berries, sesame oil, watercress, and parsley. Season with salt and black pepper, and mix well.
- ✓ Serve with lemon wedges.

72) Warm Mushroom And Orange Pepper Salad

Preparation Time: 10 minutes

Cooking Time: 8 minutes

Servings: 4

Nutrition: Calories 289, Total Fat 26.71g, Total Carbs 9g, Fiber 3.8g, Net Carbs 5.2g, Protein 4.23g

Ingredients:

- 2 tbsp avocado oil
- 1 cup mixed mushrooms, chopped
- 2 orange bell peppers, deseeded and finely sliced
- 1 garlic clove, minced
- 2 tbsp tamarind sauce
- 1 tsp maple (sugar-freesyrup
- ½ tsp hot sauce
- ½ tsp fresh ginger paste

Directions:

- ✓ Over medium fire, heat half of avocado oil in a large skillet, sauté mushroom and bell peppers until slightly softened, 5 minutes.
- ✓ In a small bowl, whisk garlic, tamarind sauce, maple syrup, hot sauce, and ginger paste. Add mixture to vegetables and stir- fry for 2 to 3 minutes.
- ✓ Turn heat off and dish salad. Drizzle with remaining avocado oil and garnish with sesame seeds.
- ✓ Serve with grilled tofu.

73) Broccoli, Kelp, And Feta Salad

Preparation Time: 15 minutes

Cooking Time:

Servings: 4

Nutrition: Calories 397, Total Fat 3.87g, Total Carbs 8.4g, Fiber 3.5g, Net Carbs 4.9g, Protein 8.93g

Ingredients:

- 2 tbsp olive oil
-
- 1 tbsp white wine vinegar
- 2 tbsp chia seeds
- Salt and freshly ground black pepper to taste
- 2 cups broccoli slaw
- 1 cup chopped kelp, thoroughly washed and steamed
- 1/3 cup chopped pecans
- 1/3 cup pumpkin seeds
- 1/3 cup blueberries
- 2/3 cup ricotta cheese

Directions:

- ✓ In a small bowl, whisk olive oil, white wine vinegar, chia seeds, salt, and black pepper. Set aside.
- ✓ In a large salad bowl, combine the broccoli slaw, kelp, pecans, pumpkin seeds, blueberries, and ricotta cheese.
- ✓ Drizzle dressing on top, toss, and serve.

74) Roasted Asparagus With Feta Cheese Salad

Preparation Time: 10 minutes

Cooking Time: 20 minutes

Servings: 4

Nutrition: Calories 146, Total Fat 12.87g, Total Carbs 5.07g, Fiber 1.6g, Net Carbs 3.47g, Protein 4.44g

Ingredients:

- 1 lb asparagus, trimmed and halved
- 2 tbsp olive oil
- ½ tsp dried basil
- ½ tsp dried oregano
- Salt and freshly ground black pepper to taste
- ½ tsp hemp seeds
- 1 tbsp maple (sugar-freesyrup
- ½ cup arugula
- 4 tbsp crumbled feta cheese
- 2 tbsp hazelnuts
- 1 lemon, cut into wedges

Directions:

- ✓ Preheat oven to 350oF.
- ✓ Pour asparagus on a baking tray, drizzle with olive oil, basil, oregano, salt, black pepper, and hemp seeds. Mix with your hands and roast in oven for 15 minutes.
- ✓ Remove, drizzle with maple syrup, and continue cooking until slightly charred, 5 minutes.
- ✓ Spread arugula in a salad bowl and top with asparagus. Scatter with feta cheese, hazelnuts, and serve with lemon wedges.

75) Spicy Broccoli Salad

Preparation Time: 45 minutes

Cooking Time:

Servings: 2

Nutrition: Carbs: 10.5 g Protein:2.6g Fats: 7.5g Calories: 133Kcal

Ingredients:

- Broccoli: 2 cups cut in big florets
- Hot sauce: 2 tbsp
- Rice vinegar: 1 tbsp
- Salt: as per your taste
- Pepper: as per your taste
- Sliced red pepper: 1 cup sliced
- Olive oil: 1 tbsp

Directions:

- ✓ Preheat the oven 200C
- ✓ Add broccoli to the baking sheet and sprinkle seasoning and brush with olive oil
- ✓ Roast for 25 minutes till it turns golden and soft
- ✓ Take a small bowl and combine hot sauce, vinegar, salt, and pepper
- ✓ Remove broccoli from oven and brush with this dressing and Cooking Time: in the oven again for 10 minutes. Serve with red pepper.

Plant Based Vegetable Recipes

76) Spinach Hummus

Preparation Time: 10 minutes

Cooking Time:

Servings: 4 as a side dish

Nutrition: Carbs: 25.8g Protein: 10.7g Fats: 18.6g Calories: 296Kcal

Ingredients:

- Chickpeas: 2 cups tin drained and rinsed
- Baby spinach: 1 cup
- Tahini: 3 tbsp
- Garlic: 1 clove
- Lemon: 2 tbsp
- Extra-virgin olive oil: 3 tbsp, plus extra to serve
- Salt: as per your need

Directions:

- ✓ Blend baby spinach, chickpeas, tahini, olive oil, salt, and garlic together in a blender
- ✓ Add in lemon juice and mix
- ✓ Add to the serving bowl and top with extra olive oil

77) Stir Fry Turmeric Butternut Squash

Preparation Time: 30 minutes

Cooking Time:

Servings: 2

Nutrition: Carbs: 22g Protein:1.9g Fats:14.2g Calories: 201Kcal

Ingredients:

- Olive oil: 2 tbsp
- Butternut squash: 2 cups
- Turmeric: 1 tsp
- Salt: as per your taste
- Red pepper: ½ tsp

Directions:

- ✓ Take a pan and heat olive oil
- ✓ Take a bowl and add butternut squash, salt, turmeric, pepper and mix well and add to the pan
- ✓ Fry on low heat for 20 minutes and turn in between
- ✓ Serve as a salad with the main dish

78) Rainbow Vegetable Bowl

Preparation Time: 25 minute

Cooking Time:

Servings: 4

Nutrition: Carbs: 29.9g Protein: 5.9g Fats: 10g Calories: 227 Kcal

Ingredients:

- Red bell Pepper: 1
- Yellow bell pepper: 1
- Smoked Paprika: ½ tsp
- Potatoes: 3 medium
- Mushrooms: 8 oz
- Yellow Onion: 1
- Zucchini: 1
- Cumin Powder: ½ tsp
- Garlic Powder: ½ tsp
- Salt and Pepper: as per your taste
- Cooking oil: 2 tbsp (optional

Directions:

- ✓ Heat a large pan on medium flame, add oil and put the sliced potatoes
- ✓ Cooking Time: the potatoes till they change color
- ✓ Cut the rest of the vegetables and add all the spices
- ✓ Cooked till veggies are soften

79) Red Bell Pepper Hummus

Preparation Time: 10 minutes

Cooking Time:

Servings: 4 as a side dish

Nutrition: Carbs: 27.1g Protein: 9.8g Fats: 18.7g Calories: 302Kcal

Ingredients:

- Chickpeas: 2 cups can rinsed and drained
- Red bell pepper: 1 cup diced
- Tahini: 3 tbsp
- Garlic: 1 clove
- Lemon: 2 tbsp
- Extra-virgin olive oil: 3 tbsp, plus extra to serve
- Salt: as per your need
- Cayenne pepper: 1 tsp

Directions:

- ✓ Chickpeas: 2 cups can rinsed and drained
- ✓ Red bell pepper: 1 cup diced
- ✓ Tahini: 3 tbsp
- ✓ Garlic: 1 clove
- ✓ Lemon: 2 tbsp
- ✓ Extra-virgin olive oil: 3 tbsp, plus extra to serve
- ✓ Salt: as per your need
- ✓ Cayenne pepper: 1 tsp

80) Simple Peas Mix

Preparation Time: 5minutes

Cooking Time:

Servings: 2

Nutrition: Carbs: 10g Protein: 5g Fats: 6.5g Calories: 133Kcal

Ingredients:

- Frozen peas: 1 cup can washed and drained
- Salt: as per your taste
- Pepper: as per your taste
- Cashew cream: ½ cup

Directions:

- ✓ Combine all the ingredients
- ✓ Serve as the side dish

81) Spinach Green Hummus

Preparation Time: 10 minutes

Cooking Time:

Servings: 4 as a side dish

Nutrition: Carbs: 34.2g Protein: 16.9g Fats:22.7g Calories: 295Kcal

Ingredients:

- Chickpeas: 2 cups drained and rinsed
- Spinach: 1 cup
- Pistachios: 1 cup finely shredded
- Tahini: 3 tbsp
- Garlic: 1 clove
- Lemon juice: 2 tbsp
- Salt: as per your need
- Sesame seed: ½ tsp
- Water: 3 tbsp

Directions:

- ✓ Blend spinach, chickpeas, tahini, water, salt, and garlic together in a blender
- ✓ Add in lemon juice and mix
- ✓ Add to the serving bowl and top with sesame seeds and pistachios

82) Stir-Fry Greens

Preparation Time: 30 minutes

Cooking Time:

Servings: 2

Nutrition: Carbs: 21.5g Protein:9.4g Fats: 9.55g Calories: 127.2Kcal Rice Milk

Ingredients:

- Long-stemmed broccoli: 1 cup
- Kale: 1 cup
- Olive oil: 1 tbsp
- Peas: 1 cup
- Salt: as per your taste
- Smoked paprika: ½ tsp

Directions:

- ✓ Take a pan and heat olive oil
- ✓ Take a bowl and add broccoli, peas, salt, paprika and mix well and add to the pan
- ✓ Fry on low heat for 20 minutes and turn in between
- ✓ Add kale at the last minutes
- ✓ Serve as a salad with the main dish

83) Overnight soaking

Preparation Time:20 minutes

Cooking Time:

Servings: 400ml

Nutrition: Carbs: 7.5g Protein: 0.4g Fats: 0.1g Calories: 33Kcal

Ingredients:

- Rice: 250g
- Maple syrup: 2 tsp
- Water: 500 ml

Directions:

- ✓ Toast rice in the pan lightly and soak overnight in 250ml water
- ✓ Add maple syrup, rice, and 250ml water to the blender and blend till smoothen
- ✓ Strain and discard the puree
- ✓ Shake before serving

84) Roasted Chili Potatoes

Preparation Time: 35 minutes

Cooking Time:

Servings: 2

Nutrition: Carbs: 26 g Protein: 3g Fats: 7.2g Calories: 178Kcal

Ingredients:

- Olive oil: 1 tbsp
- Potatoes: 2 cups cut like fries
- Salt: as per your taste
- Pepper: as per your taste
- Red chili flakes: 1 tsp

Directions:

- ✓ Preheat the oven 200C
- ✓ Add potatoes to the baking sheet and sprinkle seasoning and brush with olive oil
- ✓ Roast for 25 minutes till it turns golden and soft
- ✓ Remove from the oven and sprinkle red chili flakes
- ✓ Serve as the side dish

85) Roasted Parsnips With Zhoug

Preparation Time: 35 minutes

Cooking Time:

Servings: 4

Nutrition: Carbs: 24g Protein: 1.6g Fats: 3.9g Calories: 141Kcal

Ingredients:

- Parsnips: 4 thickly sliced
- Salt and pepper: as per your taste
- Olive oil: 1 tbsp
- For the Zhoug:
- Flat-leaf parsley: ½ cup chopped
- Coriander: ½ cup chopped
- Vinegar: 1 tbsp
- Green chili: 1 chopped
- Garlic:½ clove chopped
- Ground cumin: ½ tsp

Directions:

- ✓ Preheat the oven to 200C
- ✓ Take a baking sheet and place parsnips
- ✓ Brush oil and sprinkle salt and pepper
- ✓ Bake for 25-30 minutes till they tender
- ✓ In the meanwhile, add all the zhoug ingredients to the food processor and blend
- ✓ Add 3-4 tablespoons of water if needed
- ✓ Serve roasted parsnips with zhoug

86) Roasted Broccoli With Peanuts And Kecap Manis

Preparation Time: 40 minutes

Cooking Time:

Servings: 4

Nutrition: Carbs: 22.5 g Protein: 9.4 g Fats: 12.8 g Calories:258 Kcal

Ingredients:

- Broccoli: a large head diced
- Vegetable oil: 1 tbsp
- Kecap manis: 4 tbsp
- Spring onions: 2 sliced
- Grated garlic: 2 cloves
- Sesame oil: 2 tbsp
- Ginger: 1 tbsp grated
- Dried chili flakes: a pinch
- Salted peanuts: a handful roughly chopped
- Rice vinegar: 3 tbsp
- Coriander: ½ cup chopped
- Ready-made crispy onions: 3 tbsp
- Water: 50ml
- Cooked jasmine rice to serve

Directions:

- ✓ Preheat the oven to 180C
- ✓ Take a large pan and add oil and fry broccoli in batches and spread on baking sheet
- ✓ In the same pan, fry garlic, ginger, and chili flakes for a minute and then add rice vinegar, manis, sesame oil, and water
- ✓ Pour all of this mixture over broccoli and cover with foil
- ✓ Roast the broccoli for 20 minutes in the oven
- ✓ Mix crispy onion and salted peanuts together and sprinkle over cooked broccoli
- ✓ Top with coriander and serve with rice

87) Roasted Red Cabbage Pesto

Preparation Time: 10 minutes

Cooking Time:

Servings: 4 as a side dish

Nutrition: Carbs: 11.8g Protein: 10.4g Fats: 34.2g Calories: 366Kcal

Ingredients:

- Red cabbage: 1 head small
- Garlic: 2 cloves
- Lemon juice: 3 tbsp
- Ground almonds: 2 tbsp
- Extra-virgin olive oil: 3 tbsp
- Salt: as per your need
- Chili sauce: 1 tbsp

Directions:

- ✓ Roast cabbage in the oven for 10 minutes at 160C
- ✓ Take a blender and add all the ingredients including roasted cabbage
- ✓ Blend them well
- ✓ Serve with crispy chips

88) Roasted Garlic Toasts

Preparation Time: 45 minutes

Cooking Time:

Servings: 4

Nutrition: Protein: 8.8 g Fats: 18.2 g Calories: 358 Kcal

Ingredients:

- Whole bulbs garlic: 4
- Olive oil: 400ml
- Cherry tomatoes: 300g halved
- Sprigs thyme: 6
- Toasted sourdough: 4 slices

Directions:

- ✓ Preheat the oven to medium heat
- ✓ Cut the garlic horizontally and sprinkle thyme and salt, and add to the bowl filled with oil
- ✓ Place in the oven and Cooking Time: for 25 minutes till garlic becomes soft
- ✓ Remove from the oven and spread on the toasted sourdough
- ✓ Top with cherry tomatoes and serve

89) Roasted Olive Oil Tomatoes

Preparation Time: 1 hour 50 minutes

Cooking Time:

Servings: 5

Nutrition: Carbs: 4.6g Protein: 1.3g Fats: 33.6g Calories: 328Kcal

Ingredients:

- Cherry tomatoes on the vine: 4-6 bunches
- Bay leaves: 6
- Olive oil: 200ml
- Garlic: 1 whole bulb cut in ½
- Crusty bread warmed to serve

Directions:

- ✓ Heat the oven to 150C
- ✓ Put the garlic and tomatoes in a baking dish, now add bay leaves and season
- ✓ Pour the olive oil on a baking dish and cover it with foil
- ✓ Let it bake for 1 ½ hour and then serve it with crusty bread

90) Rocket Chickpeas Salad

Preparation Time: 15 minutes

Cooking Time:

Servings: 2

Nutrition: Carbs: 60.4g Protein: 18.3g Fats: 26.4g Calories: 586Kcal

Ingredients:

- Avocado: 1 cut into small pieces
- Chickpeas: 400g can drained and rinsed
- Red chili: 1 chopped
- Cumin seeds: 1 tsp
- Red onion: 1/2 finely chopped
- Roasted red peppers: 3 chopped
- Olive oil
- Lime: 1 plus wedges to serve
- Rocket: 2 handfuls
- Pitta bread: 2 warmed

Directions:

- ✓ Mix onion, avocado, peppers, chickpeas, and chili in a bowl
- ✓ Take two tablespoons of olive oil and whisk it with lime juice while adding seasoning and cumin seeds
- ✓ Put it in the bowl and mix well
- ✓ Add the chickpeas mixture to the rocket pile into 2 plates
- ✓ Best served with warm pittas

91) Savory Broccoli Mash

Preparation Time: 30 minutes

Cooking Time:

Servings: 4 as a side dish

Nutrition: Carbs: 5.5g Protein: 4.07g Fats: 14.5g Calories: 178Kcal

Ingredients:

- Broccoli: 2 cups florets
- Spinach: 1 cup
- Tahini: 2 tbsp
- Garlic: 1 clove
- Vinegar: 1 tbsp
- Pepper: as per your need
- Salt: as per your need

Directions:

- ✓ Broccoli: 2 cups florets
- ✓ Spinach: 1 cup
- ✓ Tahini: 2 tbsp
- ✓ Garlic: 1 clove
- ✓ Vinegar: 1 tbsp
- ✓ Pepper: as per your need
- ✓ Salt: as per your need

92) Savory Mango Chat

Preparation Time: 5 minutes

Cooking Time:

Servings: 4

Nutrition: Carbs:50 g Protein:2.8 g Fats:1.3 g Calories: 201Kcal

Ingredients:

- Mango: 4 peeled and diced into bite-sized chunks
- Chaat masala: 2 tsp
- Lime: 1 juiced
- Sea salt: ½ tsp
- Coconut yogurt to serve

Directions:

- ✓ Place all the ingredients in a large bowl and shake them well
- ✓ Now serve it with some coconut yogurt if you desire

93) Som Tam Salad

Preparation Time: 20 minutes and marinating as well

Cooking Time:

Servings: 2

Nutrition: Carbs: 20.6 g Protein: 8.9 g Fats: 5.2 g Calories: 178 Kcal

Ingredients:

- Green beans: 110g cooked and divided
- Courgettes: 2
- Cherry tomatoes: 120g halved
- Carrot: 1 shredded
- Lime: 1 juiced
- Palm sugar: 1 tbsp
- Tamari: 1 tbsp
- Coriander: ¼ cup chopped
- Mint: ¼ cup chopped
- Chili: 1 finely sliced
- Roasted peanuts: 1 tbsp chopped

Directions:

- ✓ With the spiraliser, create thin strands of courgette
- ✓ Add green beans, cherry tomatoes, carrots, lime juice, palm sugar, and chili and give pulse in the blender or crush in pestle and mortar
- ✓ Add the mixture to the courgette and mix for 15 minutes
- ✓ Top with chopped peanuts, mint, and coriander, combine well and serve

94) Steamed Brinjal With Peanut Dressing

Preparation Time: 20 minutes

Cooking Time:

Servings: 4

Nutrition: Carbs: 4.8 g Protein: 2.8 g Fats: 6.2 g Calories: 89 Kcal

Ingredients:

- Baby brinjals: 360g pack halved
- Rice vinegar: 1 tbsp
- Peanut butter: 1 tbsp
- Soy sauce: 1 tbsp
- Chilli oil: 1 tbsp
- Spring onions: 2 thinly sliced
- Caster sugar: 1 tbsp
- Sesame seeds: 2 tsp toasted
- Coriander: 2 tbsp chopped

Directions:

- ✓ Add brinjals to the steamer and steam for 15 minutes
- ✓ In a bowl, add peanut butter and a splash of boiling water then include soy sauce, sugar, vinegar, and chili oil
- ✓ Take a serving tray and place brinjals and top with the sauce
- ✓ Sprinkle sesame seeds, coriander, and spring onions from above

95) Sticky Seeds And Nuts

Preparation Time: 0 minutes

Cooking Time:

Servings: make 6 portions

Nutrition: Carbs: 25.1g

Protein: 16.1g Fats: 32.7g Calories: 462Kcal

Ingredients:

- Whole almonds: 100g
- Cashew nuts: 100g
- Black or white sesame seeds: 3 tbsp
- Black peppercorns: ¼ tsp
- Peanuts: 100g
- Granulated sugar: 100g
- Brown miso paste: 2 tbsp
- Toasted sesame oil: 2 tsp
- Pumpkin seeds: 25g
- Sunflower seeds: 25g

Directions:

- ✓ Preheat the oven to 180C
- ✓ Take a baking sheet and place the nuts
- ✓ Bake for15 minutes till they turn golden brown
- ✓ Take a pan and add sugar with 4tbsp water
- ✓ Let the sugar to melt on the low heat and stir in between
- ✓ Allow it to turn golden and remove from heat and add in sesame oil
- ✓ Add in miso while stirring gently
- ✓ Take a large bowl and add nuts, seeds, and black pepper
- ✓ Pour caramel from the top and stir continuously to coat the seeds and nuts evenly
- ✓ Line a tray with a baking paper and add nuts and seeds and allow to cool
- ✓ Divide and eat right away or store for a week in a sterilized airtight jar

96) Sweet Potato Salad With Salad And Green Dip

Preparation Time: 45 minutes

Cooking Time:

Servings: 4

Nutrition: Carbs: 55g Protein: 10g Fats: 3.7g Calories: 313Kcal

Ingredients:

- Gram flour: 120g
- Sweet potato: 1 large
- Olive oil
- Middle eastern wraps to serve
- Ground cumin: 1 tsp
- Coriander: 1 tbsp chopped
- Ginger grated to make: 1 tsp
- Garlic: 1 clove crushed
- Mild chili powder: ½ tsp
- For the Coriander Chutney
- Coriander: a bunch chopped
- Shallot: 1 small chopped
- Green chili: 1 chopped
- Ginger: a chunk peeled and chopped
- Lemon: ½ juiced
- For the Carrot Salad
- Carrots: 2 peeled and grated
- Lemon:: ½ juiced
- Cumin seeds: 1 tsp toasted
- Coriander leaves: ½ small bunch chopped

Directions:

- ✓ Heat the oven to 200C
- ✓ Prick sweet potatoes with the fork and bake for 10 minutes
- ✓ Allow to cool and add to the bowl and add the remaining falafel ingredients and mix
- ✓ Make the mixture into 12 flattish balls with your hands
- ✓ Now cover the balls with oiled baking
- ✓ sheet and let it bake for 10-15 minutes till they are dry and golden
- ✓ Add the ingredients of coriander chutney into a blender and add water if necessary, blend till its smooth then season and put in a bowl
- ✓ Put the carrot salad ingredients with some seasoning and add 1 teaspoon of oil on top
- ✓ Now serve falafels with coriander chutney, wraps, and carrot salad

97) Sweet Potato Spicy Bites

Preparation Time: 30 minutes

Cooking Time:

Servings: 4

Nutrition: Carbs: 166g

Protein: 11g Fats: 16g Calories: 211Kcal

Ingredients:

- Sweet potato: 3 peeled and sliced
- Olive oil: 1 tbsp
- Salt and pepper: as per your taste
- For the dressing:
- Lemon: 1 tsp
- Salt and pepper: as per your taste
- Vegan chipotle mayo: 2 tbsp
- Chili: 1 tbsp finely chopped
- Hot sauce: 1 tbsp
- Fresh herbs: 3 tbsp

Directions:

- ✓ Preheat the oven 200C
- ✓ Add sweet potatoes to the baking sheet and olive oil
- ✓ Roast for 25 minutes till it turns golden and soft
- ✓ Add all the dressing together and pour on to the sweet potatoes
- ✓ Serve as the side dish

98) Tarragon Cauli Salad

Preparation Time: 45 minutes

Cooking Time:

Servings: 2

Nutrition: Carbs: 3.45g Protein: 2.42g Fats: 14.22g Calories: 177.75Kcal

Ingredients:

- Cauliflower: 1 cup florets
- Salt: as per your need
- Pepper: as per your need
- Olive oil: 1 tbsp
- For The Tarragon Dressing:
- Tarragon: ½ bunch
- Baby spinach: ½ cup
- Dijon mustard: 1 tsp
- Lemon juice: 1 tbsp
- Capers: 2 tsp
- Salt: ½ tsp
- Olive oil: 2 tbsp

Directions:

- ✓ Preheat the oven to 200C
- ✓ Take a baking sheet and place cauliflower florets
- ✓ Brush oil and sprinkle salt and pepper
- ✓ Bake for 25-30 minutes till they tender
- ✓ Add all the tarragon dressing ingredients into the bowl with water
- ✓ Add to the blender and blend and make smooth and thick
- ✓ Add cauliflower to the bowl and top with the dressing
- ✓ Serve as the side dish

99) Tarragon Spinach Cauliflower Salad

Preparation Time: 45 minutes

Cooking Time:

Servings: 3

Nutrition: Carbs: 4.6g Protein: 3.23g Fats: 9.6g Calories: 105Kcal

Ingredients:

- Cauliflower: 2 cups
- olive oil: 2 tbsp
- Garlic powder: 1 tbsp
- Baby spinach: 1 cup
- Tarragon: ½ a bunch
- Salt: as per your taste
- Pepper: as per your taste
- Lemon juice: 1 tbsp

Directions:

- ✓ Preheat the oven 200C
- ✓ Add cauliflowers to the baking sheet and sprinkle seasoning and brush with olive oil
- ✓ Roast for 25 minutes till turn golden and soft
- ✓ Remove from the oven and sprinkle spinach, tarragon, salt, pepper, garlic powder, and lemon juice on top
- ✓ Serve as a side dish

100) Temaki

Preparation Time: 1 hour

Cooking Time:

Servings: 3

Nutrition: Carbs: 45.2 g Protein: 6.7 g Fats: 7.8 g Calories: 278 Kcal

Ingredients:

- Brown sushi rice: 150g
- Avocado: ½ thinly sliced
- Carrot: 1 small shredded
- Cucumber: ¼ cut into small pieces
- Rice vinegar: 1 tbsp
- Nori sheets: 3
- Roasted red pepper: 1 cut into strips
- For a Dipping Sauce:
- Red chili: ½ deseeded and chopped
- Light soy sauce: 2 tbsp
- Sesame seeds: 2 tsp toasted
- Rice vinegar: 2 ts

Directions:

- ✓ Wash the rice and drain and add into the pan with salt and water
- ✓ Boil the mixture, cover and Cooking Time: for 30 minutes
- ✓ Add in rice vinegar and stir and leave to cool for 5 minutes
- ✓ Cut nori sheets diagonally to create six triangles
- ✓ Add the rice to the triangles leaving behind the corners
- ✓ Mix carrot, cucumber, pepper, and avocado to the bowl and add to the rice
- ✓ Create cones
- ✓ Add all the ingredients of the sauce in the bowl and serve with the cones

Plant Based Main Recipes

101) Grilled tempeh with green beans

Preparation Time: 15 minutes

Cooking Time:

Servings: 4

Nutrition: Calories 352 Fats 22.5g| Carbs 21.8g Protein 22.6g

Ingredients:

- 2 tbsp olive oil
- 1½ lb tofu, cut into strips
- Salt and ground black pepper to taste
- If there is ever a dish that can replace the essence of BBQ, this would be it! Plus the extra ingredients of green beans.
- 1 tbsp plant butter, melted
- 1 lb tempeh, sliced into 4 pieces
- 1 lb green beans, trimmed
- Salt and black pepper to taste
- 2 sprigs thyme
- 2 tbsp olive oil
- 1 tbsp pure corn syrup
- 1 lemon, juiced

Directions:

- ✓ Preheat a grill pan over medium heat and brush with the plant butter.
- ✓ Season the tempeh and green beans with the salt, black pepper, and place the thyme in the pan. Grill the tempeh and green beans on both sides until golden brown and tender, 10 minutes.
- ✓ Transfer to serving plates.
- ✓ In a small bowl, whisk the olive oil, corn syrup, lemon juice, and drizzle all over the food.
- ✓ Serve warm.

102) Tofu Fajita Bowl

Preparation Time: 5minutes

Cooking Time: 10minutes

Servings: 4

Nutrition: Calories:263, Total Fat:26.4g, Saturated Fat:8.8g, Total Carbs:4g, Dietary Fiber:1g, Sugar:3g, Protein:4g, Sodium:826mg

Ingredients:

- 2 tbsp Tex-Mex seasoning
- 1 small iceberg lettuce, chopped
- 2 large tomatoes, deseeded and chopped
- 2 avocados, halved, pitted, and chopped
- 1 green bell pepper, deseeded and thinly sliced
- 1 yellow onion, thinly sliced
- 4 tbsp fresh cilantro leaves
- ½ cup shredded dairy- free parmesan cheese blend
- 1 cup plain unsweetened yogurt

Directions:

- ✓ Heat the olive oil in a medium skillet over medium heat, season the tofu with salt, black pepper, and Tex-Mex seasoning. Fry in the oil on both sides until golden and cooked, 5 to 10 minutes. Transfer to a plate.
- ✓ Divide the lettuce into 4 serving bowls, share the tofu on top, and add the tomatoes, avocados, bell pepper, onion, cilantro, and cheese.
- ✓ Top with dollops of plain yogurt and serve immediately with low carb

103) Tofu- Seitan Casserole

Preparation Time: 10minutes

Cooking Time: 20minutes

Servings: 4

Nutrition: Calories475:, Total Fat:41.2g, Saturated Fat:12.3g, Total Carbs:6g, Dietary Fiber:3g, Sugar:2g, Protein:24g, Sodium:755mg

Ingredients:

- 1 tofu, shredded
- 7 oz seitan, chopped
- 8 oz dairy- free cream cheese (vegan
- 1 tbsp Dijon mustard
- 1 tbsp plain vinegar
- 10 oz shredded cheddar cheese
- Salt and ground black pepper to taste

Directions:

- ✓ Preheat the oven to 350 F and grease a baking dish with cooking spray. Set aside.
- ✓
- ✓ Spread the tofu and seitan in the bottom of the dish.
- ✓ In a small bowl, mix the cashew cream, Dijon mustard, vinegar, and two-thirds of the cheddar cheese. Spread the mixture on top of the tofu and seitan, season with salt and black pepper, and cover with the remaining cheese.
- ✓ Bake in the oven for 15 to 20 minutes or until the cheese melts and is golden brown.
- ✓ Remove the dish and serve with steamed collards.

104) Ginger Lime Tempeh

Preparation Time: 10 minutes

Cooking Time: 40 minutes

Servings: 4

Nutrition: Calories:285, Total Fat:25.6g, Saturated Fat:13.6g, Total Carbs:7g, Dietary Fiber:2g, Sugar:2g, Protein:11g, Sodium:772mg

Ingredients:

- 5 kaffir lime leaves
- 1 tbsp cumin powder
- 1 tbsp ginger powder
- 1 cup plain unsweetened yogurt
- 2 lb tempeh
- Salt and ground black pepper to taste
- 1 tbsp olive oil
- 2 limes, juiced

Directions:

- ✓ In a large bowl, combine the kaffir lime leaves, cumin, ginger, and plain yogurt. Add the tempeh, season with salt, and black pepper, and mix to coat well. Cover the bowl with a plastic wrap and marinate in the refrigerator for 2 to 3 hours.
- ✓ Preheat the oven to 350 F and grease a baking sheet with cooking spray.
- ✓ Take out the tempeh and arrange on the baking sheet. Drizzle with olive oil, lime juice, cover with aluminum foil, and slow- Cooking Time: in the oven for 1 to 1 ½ hours or until the tempeh cooks within.
- ✓ Remove the aluminum foil, turn the broiler side of the oven on, and brown the top of the tempeh for 5 to 10 minutes.
- ✓ Take out the tempeh and serve warm with red cabbage slaw.

105) Tofu Mozzarella

Preparation Time: 10minutes

Cooking Time: 35minutes

Servings: 4

Nutrition: Calories:140, Total Fat:13.2g, Saturated Fat:7.1g, Total Carbs:2g, Dietary Fiber:0g, Sugar:0g, Protein:3g, Sodium:78mg1

Ingredients:

- 1½ lb tofu, halved lengthwise
- Salt and ground black pepper to taste
- 2 eggs
- 2 tbsp Italian seasoning
- 1 pinch red chili flakes
- ½ cup sliced Pecorino Romano cheese
- ¼ cup fresh parsley, chopped
- 4 tbsp butter
- 2 garlic cloves, minced
- 2 cups crushed tomatoes
- 1 tbsp dried basil
- Salt and ground black pepper to taste
- ½ lb sliced mozzarella cheese

Directions:

- ✓ Preheat the oven to 400 F and grease a baking dish with cooking spray. Set aside.
- ✓ Season the tofu with salt and black pepper; set aside.
- ✓ In a medium bowl, whisk the eggs with the Italian seasoning, and red chili flakes. In a plate, combine the Pecorino Romano cheese with parsley.
- ✓ Melt the butter in a medium skillet over medium heat.
- ✓ Quickly dip the tofu in the egg mixture and then dredge generously in the cheese mixture. Place in the butter and fry on both sides until the cheese melts and is golden brown, 8 to 10 minutes. Place on a plate and set aside.
- ✓ Sauté the garlic in the same pan and mix in the tomatoes. Top with the basil, salt, and black pepper, and Cooking Time: for 5 to 10 minutes. Pour the sauce into the baking dish.
- ✓ Lay the tofu pieces in the sauce and top with the mozzarella cheese. Bake in the oven for 10 to 15 minutes or until the cheese melts completely.
- ✓ Remove the dish and serve with leafy green salad.

106) Seitan Meatza With Kale

Preparation Time: 10minutes

Cooking Time: 22minutes

Servings: 4

Nutrition: Calories:601, Total Fat:51.8g, Saturated Fat:16.4g, Total Carbs:18g, Dietary Fiber:5g, Sugar:3g, Protein:23g, Sodium:398mg

Ingredients:

- 1 lb ground seitan
- Salt and black pepper to taste
- 2 cups powdered Parmesan cheese
- ¼ tsp onion powder
- ¼ tsp garlic powder
- ½ cup unsweetened tomato sauce
- 1 tsp white vinegar
- ½ tsp liquid smoke
- ¼ cup baby kale, chopped roughly
- 1 cup mozzarella cheese

Directions:

- ✓ Preheat the oven to 400 F and line a medium pizza pan with parchment paper and grease with cooking spray. Set aside.
- ✓ In a medium bowl, combine the seitan, salt, black pepper, and parmesan cheese. Spread the mixture on the pizza pan to fit the shape of the pan. Bake in the oven for 15 minutes or until the meat cooks.
- ✓ Meanwhile in a medium bowl, mix the onion powder, garlic powder, tomato sauce, vinegar, and liquid smoke. Remove the meat crust from the oven and spread the tomato mixture on top. Add the kale and sprinkle with the mozzarella cheese.
- ✓ Bake in the oven for 7 minutes or until the cheese melts.
- ✓ Take out from the oven, slice, and serve warm.

107) Taco Tempeh Casserole

Preparation Time: 10minutes

Cooking Time: 20minutes

Servings: 4

Nutrition: Calories:132, Total Fat:11.5g, Saturated Fat4:4.3g, Total Carbs:7g, Dietary Fiber:4g, Sugar:2g, Protein:1g, Sodium:10mg

Ingredients:

- 1 Tempeh, shredded
- 1/3 cup vegan mayonnaise
- 8 oz dairy- free cream cheese (vegan
- 1 yellow onion, sliced
- 1 yellow bell pepper, deseeded and chopped
- 2 tbsp taco seasoning
- ½ cup shredded cheddar cheese
- Salt and ground black pepper to taste

Directions:

- ✓ Preheat the oven to 400 F and grease a baking dish with cooking spray.
- ✓ Into the dish, put the tempeh, mayonnaise, cashew cream, onion, bell pepper, taco seasoning, and two-thirds of the cheese, salt, and black pepper. Mix the Ingredients and top with the remaining cheese.
- ✓ Bake in the oven for 15 to 20 minutes or until the cheese melts and is golden brown.
- ✓ Remove the dish, plate, and serve with lettuce leaves.

108) Broccoli Tempeh Alfredo

Preparation Time: 10minutes

Cooking Time: 15minutes

Servings: 4

Nutrition: Calories:193, Total Fat:20.1g, Saturated Fat:12.5g, Total Carbs:3g, Dietary Fiber:0g, Sugar:2g, Protein:1g, Sodium:100mg

Ingredients:

- 6 slices tempeh, chopped
- 2 tbsp butter
- 4 tofu, cut into 1-inch cubes
- Salt and ground black pepper to taste
- 4 garlic cloves, minced
- 1 cup baby kale, chopped
- 1 ½ cups full- fat heavy creaminutes
- 1 medium head broccoli, cut into florets
- ¼ cup shredded parmesan cheese

Directions:

- ✓ Put the tempeh in a medium skillet over medium heat and fry until crispy and brown, 5 minutes. Spoon onto a plate and set aside.
- ✓ Melt the butter in the same skillet, season the tofu with salt and black pepper, and Cooking Time: on both sides until goldern- brown. Spoon onto the tempeh's plate and set aside.
- ✓ Add the garlic to the skillet, sauté for 1 minute.
- ✓ Mix in the full- fat heavy cream, tofu, and tempeh, and kale, allow simmering for 5 minutes or until the sauce thickens.
- ✓ Meanwhile, pour the broccoli into a large safe-microwave bowl, sprinkle with some water, season with salt, and black pepper, and microwave for 2 minutes or until the broccoli softens.
- ✓ Spoon the broccoli into the sauce, top with the parmesan cheese, stir and Cooking Time: until the cheese melts. Turn the heat off. Serve warm.

109) Seitan Mushroom Burgers

Preparation Time: 15 minutes

Cooking Time: 13 minutes

Servings: 4

Nutrition: Calories:304, Total Fat:29g, Saturated Fat:23.5g, Total Carbs:8g, Dietary Fiber:3g, Sugar:1g, Protein:8g, Sodium:8mg

Ingredients:

- 1 ½ lb ground seitan
- Salt and ground black pepper to taste
- 1 tbsp unsweetened tomato sauce
- 6 large Portobello caps, destemmed
- 1 tbsp olive oil
- 6 slices cheddar cheese
- For topping:
- 4 lettuce leaves
- 4 large tomato slices
- ¼ cup mayonnaise

Directions:

- ✓ In a medium bowl, combine the seitan, salt, black pepper, and tomato sauce. Using your hands, mold the mixture into 4 patties, and set aside.
- ✓ Rinse the mushrooms under running water and pat dry.
- ✓ Heat the olive oil in a medium skillet; place in the Portobello caps and Cooking Time: until softened, 3 to 4 minutes. Transfer to a serving plate and set aside.
- ✓ Put the seitan patties in the skillet and fry on both sides until brown and compacted, 8 minutes. Place the vegan cheddar slices on the food, allow melting for 1 minute and lift each patty onto each mushroom cap.
- ✓ Divide the lettuce on top, then the tomato slices, and add some mayonnaise.
- ✓ Serve immediately.

110) Taco Tempeh Stuffed Peppers

Preparation Time: 15 minutes

Cooking Time: 41 minutes

Servings: 6

Nutrition: Calories:251, Total Fat:22.5g, Saturated Fat:3.8g, Total Carbs:13g, Dietary Fiber:9g, Sugar:2g, Protein:3g, Sodium:23mg

Ingredients:

- 6 yellow bell peppers, halved and deseeded
- 1 ½ tbsp olive oil
- Salt and ground black pepper to taste
- 3 tbsp butter
- 3 garlic cloves, minced
- ½ white onion, chopped
- 2 lbs. ground tempeh
- 3 tsp taco seasoning
- 1 cup riced broccoli
- ¼ cup grated cheddar cheese
- Plain unsweetened yogurt for serving

Directions:

- ✓ Preheat the oven to 400 F and grease a baking dish with cooking spray. Set aside.
- ✓ Drizzle the bell peppers with the olive oil and season with some salt. Set aside.
- ✓ Melt the butter in a large skillet and sauté the garlic and onion for 3 minutes. Stir in the tempeh, taco seasoning, salt, and black pepper. Cooking Time: until the meat is no longer pink, 8 minutes.
- ✓ Mix in the broccoli until adequately incorporated. Turn the heat off.
- ✓ Spoon the mixture into the peppers, top with the cheddar cheese, and place the peppers in the baking dish. Bake in the oven until the cheese melts and is bubbly, 30 minutes.
- ✓ Remove the dish from the oven and plate the peppers. Top with the palin yogurt and serve warm.

111) Vegan Bacon Wrapped Tofu With Buttered Spinach

Preparation Time: 5 minutes

Cooking Time: 20 minutes

Servings: 4

Nutrition: Calories:260, Total Fat:24.7g, Saturated Fat:14.3g, Total Carbs:4g, Dietary Fiber:0g, Sugar:2g, Protein:6g, Sodium:215mg

Ingredients:

- For the bacon wrapped tofu:
- 4 tofu
- 8 slices vegan bacon
- Salt and black pepper to taste
-
- 2 tbsp olive oil
- For the buttered spinach:
- 2 tbsp butter
- 1 lb spinach
- 4 garlic cloves
- Salt and ground black pepper to taste

Directions:

- ✓ For the bacon wrapped tofu:
- ✓ Preheat the oven to 450 F.
- ✓ Wrap each tofu with two vegan bacon slices, season with salt and black pepper, and place on the baking sheet. Drizzle with the olive oil and bake in the oven for 15 minutes or until the vegan bacon browns and the tofu cooks within.
- ✓ For the buttered spinach:
- ✓ Meanwhile, melt the butter in a large skillet, add and sauté the spinach and garlic until the leaves wilt, 5 minutes. Season with salt and black pepper.
- ✓ Serve with the buttered spinach.

112) Veggie & Tofu Kebabs

Preparation Time: 15 minutes

Cooking Time: 12 minutes

Servings: 4

Nutrition: Calories 58 Total Fat 2 g Saturated Fat 0 g Cholesterol 0 mg Sodium 84 mg Total Carbohydrate 9 g Dietary Fiber 2 g Total Sugars 5 g Protein 2 g Potassium 509 mg

Ingredients:

- 2 cloves garlic, minced
- ¼ cup balsamic vinegar
- ¼ cup olive oil
- 1 tablespoon Italian seasoning
- Salt and pepper to taste
- 1 onion, sliced into quarters
- 12 medium mushrooms
- 16 cherry tomatoes
- 1 zucchini, sliced into rounds
- 1 cup tofu, cubed
- 4 cups cauliflower rice

Directions:

- ✓ In a bowl, mix the garlic, vinegar, oil, Italian seasoning, salt and pepper.
- ✓ Toss the vegetable slices and tofu in the mixture.
- ✓ Marinate for 1 hour.
- ✓ Thread into 8 skewers and grill for 12 minutes, turning once or twice.
- ✓ Add cauliflower rice into 4 food containers.
- ✓ Add 2 kebab skewers on top of each container of cauliflower rice.
- ✓ Reheat kebabs in the grill before serving.

113) Carrot And Radish Slaw With Sesame Dressing

Preparation Time: 10 minutes

Cooking Time: 0 minute

Servings: 4

Nutrition: Calories 98 Total Fat 8 g Saturated Fat 1 g Cholesterol 0 mg Sodium 336 mg Total Carbohydrate 6 g Dietary Fiber 2 g Total Sugars 3 g Protein 2 g Potassium 241 mg

Ingredients:

- 2 tablespoons sesame oil, toasted
- 3 tablespoons rice vinegar
- ½ teaspoon sugar
- 2 tablespoons low sodium tamari
- 1 cup carrots, sliced into strips
- 2 cups radishes, sliced
- 2 tablespoons fresh cilantro, chopped
- 2 teaspoons sesame seeds, toasted

Directions:

- ✓ Mix the oil, vinegar, sugar and tamari in a bowl.
- ✓ Add the carrots, radishes and cilantro.
- ✓ Toss to coat evenly.
- ✓ Let sit for 10 minutes.
- ✓ Transfer to a food container.

114) Roasted Veggies In Lemon Sauce

Preparation Time: 15 minutes

Cooking Time: 20 minutes

Servings: 5

Nutrition: Calories 52 Total Fat 3 g Saturated Fat 0 g Cholesterol 0 mg Sodium 134 mg Total Carbohydrate 5 g Dietary Fiber 2 g Total Sugars 2 g Protein 2 g Potassium 270 mg

Ingredients:

- 2 cloves garlic, sliced
- 1 ½ cups broccoli florets
- 1 ½ cups cauliflower florets
- 1 tablespoon olive oil
- Salt to taste
- 1 teaspoon dried oregano, crushed
- ¾ cup zucchini, diced
- ¾ cup red bell pepper, diced
- 2 teaspoons lemon zest

Directions:

- ✓ Preheat your oven to 425 degrees F.
- ✓ In a baking pan, add the garlic, broccoli and cauliflower.
- ✓ Toss in oil and season with salt and oregano.
- ✓ Roast in the oven for 10 minutes.
- ✓ Add the zucchini and bell pepper to the pan.
- ✓ Stir well.
- ✓ Roast for another 10 minutes.
- ✓ Sprinkle lemon zest on top before serving.
- ✓ Transfer to a food container and reheat before serving.

115) Lunch Recipes

Preparation Time:

Cooking Time: 10 minutes

Servings: 4

Nutrition: Calories 232 Total Fat 2.1g Total Carbohydrate 44.2g

Ingredients:

- 4 whole-wheat tortillas
- 2 potatoes, boiled, cubed
- 200g refried beans
- 1 teaspoon chili powder
- ½ teaspoon dried oregano
- ¼ teaspoon garlic powder
- 120g spinach
- 1 onion, thinly sliced
- 2 cloves garlic, minced
- 30ml tamari sauce
- 45g nutritional yeast
- Salt and pepper, to taste

Directions:

- ✓ Heat a splash of olive oil in a skillet.
- ✓ Add onion and Cooking Time: over medium heat for 10 minutes, or until the onion is caramelized.
- ✓ Add the garlic and Cooking Time: 1 minute.
- ✓ Add spinach and toss gently.
- ✓ Add tamari sauce and Cooking Time: 1 minutes.
- ✓ Reheat the refried beans with nutritional yeast, chili, oregano, and garlic powder, in a microwave, on high for 1 minute.
- ✓ Mash the potatoes and spread over tortilla.
- ✓ Top the mashed potatoes with spinach mixture and refried beans.
- ✓ Season to taste and place another tortilla on top.
- ✓ Heat large skillet over medium-high heat.
- ✓ Heat the tortilla until crispy. Flip and heat the other side.
- ✓ Cut the tortilla in half and serve.

116) Lemon Pepper Pasta

Preparation Time: 5 minutes

Cooking Time: 20 minutes

Servings: 4

Nutrition: Calories 489 Total Fat 23g Total Carbohydrate 53.5g Dietary Fiber 5.9g Total Sugars 2.4g Protein 20.4g

Ingredients:

- 300g pasta, any kind, without eggs
- 400ml unsweetened soy milk
- 100g soy cream cheese
- 45g blanched almonds
- 45g nutritional yeast
- 1 teaspoon lemon zest, finely grated
- ¼ teaspoon lemon pepper
- 30ml olive oil
- 2 clove garlic, minced
- 5 capers, rinsed, chopped
- 10g parsley, chopped

Directions:

- ✓ Cooking Time: the pasta, according to the package directions, in a pot filled with salted boiling water.
- ✓ Strain the pasta and reserve 230ml cooking liquid.
- ✓ Combine soy milk, soy cheese, almonds, nutritional yeast, lemon zest, and pepper lemon in a food blender.
- ✓ Blend until smooth. Place aside.
- ✓ Heat olive oil in a skillet.
- ✓ Add the garlic, and Cooking Time: until very fragrant, for 1 minute.
- ✓ Pour in the soy milk mixture and reserved pasta cooking liquid.
- ✓ Bring to a boil, and reduce heat.
- ✓ Stir in chopped capers and simmer 6-8 minutes or until creamy. Remove from the heat and stir in cooked pasta.
- ✓ Toss the pasta gently to coat with the sauce.
- ✓ Serve pasta, garnished with chopped
- ✓
- ✓ parsley.

117) Spanish Chickpea Spinach Stew

Preparation Time: 10 minutes

Cooking Time: 25 minutes

Servings: 4

Nutrition: Calories 369 Total Fat 9.7g Total Carbohydrate 67.9g Dietary Fiber 19.9g Total Sugars 13.9g Protein 18g

Ingredients:

- 1 splash olive oil
- 1 small onion, chopped
- 2 cloves garlic
- 5g cumin powder
- 5g smoked paprika
- ¼ teaspoon chili powder
- 235ml water
- 670g can diced tomatoes
- 165g cooked chickpeas (or can chickpeas
- 60g baby spinach
- Salt, to taste
- A handful of chopped coriander, to garnish
- 20g slivered almonds, to garnish
- 4 slices toasted whole-grain bread, to serve
- with

Directions:

- ✓ Heat olive oil in a saucepan over medium- high heat.
- ✓ Add onion and Cooking Time: until browned, for 7-8 minutes.
- ✓ Add garlic, cumin, paprika, and chili powder.
- ✓ Cooking Time: 1 minute.
- ✓ Add water and scrape any browned bits.
- ✓ Add the tomatoes and chickpeas. Season to taste and reduce heat.
- ✓ Simmer the soup for 10 minutes.
- ✓ Stir in spinach and Cooking Time: 2 minutes.
- ✓ Ladle soup in a bowl. Sprinkle with cilantro and almonds.
- ✓ Serve with toasted bread slices.

118) Lentils Bolognese With Soba Noodles

Preparation Time: 10 minutes

Cooking Time: 15 minutes (plus 25 for lentils

Servings: 4

Nutrition: Calories 353 Total Fat 0.9g Total Carbohydrate 74g Dietary Fiber 9g Total Sugars 4.2g Protein 17.7g

Ingredients:

- Bolognese:
- 100g red lentils
- 1 bay leaf
- Splash of olive oil
- 1 small onion, diced
- 1 large stalk celery, sliced
- 3 cloves garlic, minced
- 230ml tomato sauce or fresh pureed tomatoes
- 60ml red wine or vegetable stock (if you do not like wine
- 1 tablespoon fresh basil, chopped
- Salt and pepper, to taste
- Soba noodles:
- 280g soba noodles

Directions:

- ✓ Cooking Time: the lentils; place lentils and bay leaf in a saucepan.
- ✓ Cover with water, so the water is 2-inches above the lentils.
- ✓ Bring to a boil over medium-high heat.
- ✓ Reduce heat and simmer the lentils for 25 minutes.
- ✓ Drain the lentils and discard the bay leaf.
- ✓ Heat a splash of olive oil in a saucepan.
- ✓ Add onion, and Cooking Time: 6 minutes.
- ✓ Add celery and Cooking Time: 2 minutes.
- ✓ Add garlic and Cooking Time: 2 minutes.
- ✓ Add the tomatoes and wine. Simmer the mixture for 5 minutes.
- ✓ Stir in the lentils and simmer 2 minutes.
- ✓ Remove the Bolognese from the heat and stir in basil.
- ✓ In the meantime, Cooking Time: the soba noodles according to package directions.
- ✓ Serve noodles with lentils Bolognese.

119) Red Burgers

Preparation Time: 10 minutes

Cooking Time: 50 minutes

Servings: 4

Nutrition: Calories 343 Total Fat 16.6g Total Carbohydrate 49.1g Dietary Fiber 14.4g Total Sugars 8.1g Protein 15g

Ingredients:

- Patties:
-
- 2 large beets, peeled, cubed
- 1 red onion, cut into chunks
- 115g red kidney beans
- 85g red cooked quinoa
- 2 cloves garlic, minced
- 30g almond meal
- 20g ground flax
- 10ml lemon juice
- ½ teaspoon ground cumin
- ½ teaspoon red pepper flakes
- Salt, to taste
- 4 whole-meal burger buns
- Tahini Guacamole:
- 1 avocado, pitted, peeled
- 45ml lime juice
- 30g tahini sauce
- 5g chopped coriander

Directions:

- ✓ Preheat oven to 190C/375F.
- ✓ Toss beet and onion with a splash of olive oil.
- ✓ Season with salt. Bake the beets for 30 minutes.
- ✓ Transfer the beets and onion into a food blender.
- ✓ Add the beans and blend until coarse. You do not want a completely smooth mixture.
- ✓ Stir in quinoa, garlic, almond meal, flax seeds, lemon juice, cumin, and red pepper flakes.
- ✓ Shape the mixture into four patties.
- ✓ Transfer the patties to a baking sheet, lined with parchment paper.
- ✓ Bake the patties 20 minutes, flipping halfway through.
- ✓ In the meantime, make the tahini guac; mash the avocado with lime juice in a bowl.
- ✓ Stir in tahini and coriander. Season to taste.
- ✓ To serve; place the patty in the bun, top with guacamole and serve.

120) Hemp Falafel With Tahini Sauce

Preparation Time: 10 minutes

Cooking Time: 10 minutes

Servings: 6

Nutrition: Calories 347 Total Fat 29.9g Total Carbohydrate 7.2g Dietary Fiber 4.3g Total Sugars 0.2g Protein 13.8g

Ingredients:

- 80g raw hemp hearts
- 4g chopped cilantro
- 4g chopped basil
- 2 cloves garlic, minced
- 2g ground cumin seeds
- 3g chili powder
- 14g flax meal + 30ml filtered water
- Sea salt and pepper, to taste
- Avocado or coconut oil, to fry
- Sauce:
- 115g tahini
- 60ml fresh lime juice
- 115ml filtered water
- 30ml extra-virgin olive oil
- Sea salt, to taste
- A good pinch ground cumin seeds

Directions:

- ✓ Mix flax with filtered water in a small bowl.
- ✓ Place aside for 10 minutes.
- ✓ In meantime, combine raw hemp hearts, cilantro, basil, garlic, cumin, chili, and seasonings in a food processor.
- ✓ Process until just comes together. Add the flax seeds mixture and process until finely blended and uniform.
- ✓ Heat approximately 2 tablespoons avocado oil in a skillet. Shape 1 tablespoon mixture into balls and fry for 3-4 minutes or until deep golden brown.
- ✓ Remove from the skillet and place on a plate lined with paper towels.
- ✓ Make the sauce; combine all ingredients in a food blender. Blend until smooth and creamy.
- ✓ Serve falafel with fresh lettuce salad and tahini sauce.

121) Tempeh Skewers With Dressing

Preparation Time: 20 minutes

Cooking Time: 10 minutes

Servings: 6

Nutrition: Calories 351 Total Fat 29.3g Total Carbohydrate 9.9g Dietary Fiber 1g Total Sugars 0.2g Protein 15.5g

Ingredients:

- 445g tempeh, cut into fingers
- 155ml unsweetened almond milk
- 100g almond flour
- 8g paprika
- 4g garlic powder
- 3g dried basil
- Salt and pepper, to taste
- 15ml olive oil
- Finger sauce:
- 60ml melted coconut oil
- 80g hot sauce
- 10 drops Stevia
- Dressing:
- 230g vegan mayonnaise
- 115g vegan sour cream
- 1 clove garlic, minced
- 2g chopped dill
- 2g chopped chives
- 1g onion powder
- Salt and pepper, to taste

Directions:

- ✓ Cut the tempeh into slices/fingers. Arrange onto bamboo skewers, soaked in water 30 minutes.
- ✓ Bring a pot of water to a boil. Add tempeh and boil 15 minutes. Drain and place aside.
- ✓ Heat oven to 200C/400F.
- ✓ Pour almond milk into a bowl. Combine almond flour and spices into a separate bowl.
- ✓ Dip the tempeh into almond milk, and coat with the almond flour mixture.
- ✓ Grease baking sheet with coconut oil. Arrange the tempeh fingers onto a baking sheet.
- ✓ Bake the tempeh 10 minutes. In the meantime, make the sauce.
- ✓ Melt coconut oil in a saucepan. Add hot sauce and simmer 5minutes. Add Stevia and remove from the heat.
- ✓ Make the dressing by combining all ingredients together.
- ✓ Toss the tempeh with hot sauce. Serve with prepared dressing.

122) White Bean Salad With Spicy Sauce

Preparation Time: 15 minutes

Cooking Time:

Servings: 4

Nutrition: Calories 366 Total Fat 24.2g Total Carbohydrate 31.9g Dietary Fiber 9.5g Total Sugars 5.6g Protein 11g

Ingredients:

- 450g can white beans, rinsed, drained or cooked beans
- 1 avocado, peeled, chopped
- 6 cherry tomatoes, quartered
- 1 red onion, thinly sliced
- Sauce:
- 80g cashews, soaked in water 4 hours
- 30ml extra-virgin olive oil
- 30ml lemon juice
- 70ml water
- 10g Dijon mustard
- 5g pure maple syrup
- 1 clove garlic
- ½ teaspoon cayenne pepper
- ½ teaspoon paprika powder
- 1 pinch salt

Directions:

- ✓ Make the sauce; rinse and drain cashews and place in a food processor.
- ✓ Add the remaining ingredients, olive oil, lemon juice, water, mustard, garlic, cayenne, paprika, and salt.
- ✓ Process until smooth and creamy. Place aside.
- ✓ Make the salad; prepared vegetables as described.
- ✓ Toss the beans with avocado, cherry tomatoes, and red onion.
- ✓ Drizzle with prepared dressing and toss once again.
- ✓ Serve or refrigerate before serving.

123) Crusted Tofu Steaks With Caramelized Onion

Preparation Time: 15 minutes

Cooking Time: 45 minutes

Servings: 4

Nutrition: Calories 617 Total Fat 29.5g Total Carbohydrate 70.6g Dietary Fiber 5.8g Total Sugars 17g Protein 23.6g

Ingredients:

- 450g tofu, cut into 8 steaks/slices
- 100g graham crackers
- 80g raw cashews
- 230ml unsweetened soy milk
- 120g whole-wheat flour
- 10g garlic powder
- 10g onion powder
- 10g chili powder
- 5g lemon pepper
- 15ml olive oil
- Salt, to taste
- Onion:
- 15ml grapeseed oil
- 1 large onion
- 15ml balsamic vinegar
- 15ml lemon juice
- 15ml water
- 15g maple sugar

Directions:

- ✓ Make the tofu; preheat oven to 200C/400F and line a baking sheet with parchment paper.
- ✓ Combine graham crackers and cashews in a food processor.
- ✓ Process unto coarse crumbs form.
- ✓ Transfer to a large bowl.
- ✓ In a separate bowl, combine flour, garlic and onion powder, chili, and lemon pepper.
- ✓ Pour the soy milk into a third bowl.
- ✓ Coat tofu with flour, dip into milk and finally coat with the graham cracker crumbs.
- ✓ Arrange the tofu steaks onto a baking sheet.
- ✓ Bake the tofu for 15-20 minutes or until golden brown.
- ✓ In the meantime, make the onion; heat grapeseed oil in a skillet.
- ✓ Add onion and Cooking Time: over medium-high heat for 8 minutes.
- ✓ Add balsamic, lemon juice, and maple sugar. Cooking Time: 2 minutes.
- ✓ Add water and reduce heat. Simmer 15 minutes.
- ✓ Serve tofu steaks with caramelized onions.

124) Spicy Beans And Rice

Preparation Time: 10 minutes

Cooking Time: 1 hour 10 minutes

Servings: 6

Nutrition: Calories 469 Total Fat 6g Total Carbohydrate 87.5g Dietary Fiber 14.2g Total Sugars 4.9g Protein 21.1g

Ingredients:

- 450g dry red kidney beans, soaked overnight
- 15ml olive oil
- 1 onion, diced
- 1 red bell pepper, seeded, diced
- 1 large stalk celery, sliced
- 4 cloves garlic, minced
- 15ml hot sauce
- 5g paprika
- 2g dried thyme
- 2 g parsley, chopped
- 2 bay leaves
- 900ml vegetable stock
- 280g brown rice
- Salt and pepper, to taste

Directions:

- ✓ Drain the beans and place aside.
- ✓ Heat olive oil in a saucepot.
- ✓ Add onion and bell pepper. Cooking Time: 6 minutes.
- ✓ Add celery and Cooking Time: 3 minutes.
- ✓ Add garlic, hot sauce, paprika, and thyme. Cooking Time: 1 minute.
- ✓ Add the drained beans, bay leaves, and vegetable stock.
- ✓ Bring to a boil, and reduce heat.
- ✓ Simmer the beans for 1 hour 15 minutes or until tender.
- ✓ In the meantime, place rice in a small saucepot. Cover the rice with 4cm water.
- ✓ Season to taste and Cooking Time: the rice until tender, for 25 minutes.
- ✓ To serve; transfer ¼ of the beans into a food processor. Process until smooth.
- ✓ Combine the processed beans with the remaining beans and ladle into a bowl.
- ✓ Add rice and sprinkle with parsley before serving.

125) Chili Quinoa Stuffed Peppers

Preparation Time: 15 minutes

Cooking Time: 1 hour 5 minutes

Servings: 4

Nutrition: Calories 456 Total Fat 15.4g Total Carbohydrate 71.1g Dietary Fiber 15.8g Total Sugars 8.2g

Ingredients:

- 160g quinoa
- 460ml vegetable stock
- 2 red bell peppers, cut in half, seeds and membrane removed
- 2 yellow bell peppers, cut in half, seeds, and membrane removed
- 120g salsa
- 15g nutritional yeast
- 10g chili powder
- 5g cumin powder
- 425g can black beans, rinsed, drained
- 160g fresh corn kernels
- Salt and pepper, to taste
- 1 small avocado, sliced
- 15g chopped cilantro

Directions:

✓ Preheat oven to 190C/375F.

✓ Brush the baking sheet with some cooking oil.

✓ Combine quinoa and vegetable stock in a saucepan. Bring to a boil.

✓ Reduce heat and simmer 20 minutes.

✓ Transfer the quinoa to a large bowl.

✓ Stir in salsa, nutritional yeast, chili powder, cumin powder, black beans, and corn. Season to taste with salt and pepper.

✓ Stuff the bell pepper halves with prepared mixture.

✓ Transfer the peppers onto a baking sheet, cover with aluminum foil, and bake for 30 minutes.

✓ Increase heat to 200C/400F and bake the peppers for an additional 15 minutes.

✓ Serve warm, topped with avocado slices, and chopped cilantro.

Plant Based Drinks & Smoothie Recipes

126) Sweet Coffee and Cacao Smoothie

Preparation Time: 3 minutes

Cooking Time:

Servings:2

Nutrition: Calories 614, Total Fat 43.2g, Saturated Fat 34.6g, Cholesterol 10mg, Sodium 146mg, Total Carbohydrate 44.7g, Dietary Fiber 5.4g, Total Sugars 31.2g, Protein 17.6g, Vitamin D 0mcg, Calcium 104mg, Iron 4mg, Potassium 614mg

Ingredients:

- 2 tsp Coffee
- ½ a Banana
- 1 cup Almond Milk
- 1 tsp Cashew Butter
- 2 tsp Cacao Powder
- 1 tsp maple Syrup
- 1 scoop vegan protein powder
- ½ cup Chocolate

Directions:

- ✓ Pop everything in a blender and blitz
- ✓ Pour into glasses and serve.

127) Amazing Blueberry Smoothie

Preparation Time: 5 minutes

Cooking Time:

Servings:2

Nutrition: Calories 269, Total Fat 12.3g, Saturated Fat 2.3g, Cholesterol 0mg, Sodium 312mg, Total Carbohydrate 37.6g, Dietary Fiber 8.2g, Total Sugars 22.9g, Protein 6.4g, Vitamin D 0mcg, Calcium 52mg, Iron 3mg, Potassium 528mg

Ingredients:

- ½ avocado
- 1 cup frozen blueberries
- 1 cup raw spinach
- ¼ tsp sea salt
- 1 cup soy
- 1 frozen banana

Directions:

- ✓ Blend everything in a powerful blender until you have a smooth, creamy shake.
- ✓ Enjoy your healthy shake and start your
- ✓ morning on a fresh note!

128) Creamy Chocolate Shake

Preparation Time: 10 minutes

Cooking Time:

Servings: 2

Nutrition: Calories 272, Total Fat 14.3g, Saturated Fat 1.5g, Cholesterol 0mg, Sodium 315mg, Total Carbohydrate 37g, Dietary Fiber 7.3g, Total Sugars 16.8g, Protein 6.2g, Vitamin D 2mcg, Calcium 735mg, Iron 2mg, Potassium 732mg

Ingredients:

- 2 frozen ripe bananas, chopped
- 1/3 cup frozen strawberries
- 2 tbsp cocoa powder
- 2 tbsp salted almond butter
- 2 cups unsweetened vanilla almond milk
- 1 dash Stevia or agave nectar
- 1/3 cup ice

Directions:

- ✓ Add all ingredients in a blender and blend until smooth.
- ✓ Take out and serve.

129) Hidden Kale Smoothie

Preparation Time: 5 minutes

Cooking Time:

Servings: 2

Nutrition: Calories 164, Total Fat 2g, Saturated Fat 0.2g, Cholesterol 0mg, Sodium 51mg, Total Carbohydrate 34.2g, Dietary Fiber 3.9g, Total Sugars 17.7g, Protein 4.1g, Vitamin D 0mcg, Calcium 124mg, Iron 2mg, Potassium 776mg

Ingredients:

- 1 medium ripe banana, peeled and sliced
- ½ cup frozen mixed berries
- 1 tbsp hulled hemp seeds
- 2 cups frozen or fresh kale
- 2/3 cup 100% pomegranate juice
- 2¼ cups filtered water

Directions:

1. Add all ingredients in a blender and blend until smooth.
2. Take out and serve.

130) Raspberry Lime Smoothie

Preparation Time: 5 minutes

Cooking Time:

Servings: 2

Nutrition: Calories 227,Total Fat 4g, Saturated Fat 1.3g, Cholesterol 0mg, Sodium 7mg, Total Carbohydrate 47.8g, Dietary Fiber 6g, Total Sugars 40.7g, Protein 0.9g, Vitamin D 0mcg, Calcium 22mg, Iron 1mg, Potassium 144mg

Ingredients:

- 1 cup water
- 1 cup fresh or frozen raspberries
- 1 large frozen banana
- 2 tbsp fresh juice, lime
- 1 tsp oil, coconut
- 1 tsp agave

Directions:

- ✓ In a blender put all ingredients and blend until smooth.
- ✓ Take out and serve

131) Peppermint Monster Smoothie

Preparation Time: 5 minutes

Cooking Time:

Servings: 1

Nutrition: Calories 799, Total Fat 28.1g, Saturated Fat 16.7g, Cholesterol 110mg, Sodium 645mg, Total Carbohydrate 98.4g, Dietary Fiber 4.5g, Total Sugars 77.2g, Protein 46.2g, Vitamin D 7mcg, Calcium 1634mg, Iron 2mg, Potassium 1366mg

Ingredients:

- 1 large frozen banana, peeled
- 1½ cups non-dairy milk
- A handful of fresh mint leaves, stems removed
- 1-2 handfuls spinach

Directions:

- ✓ In a blender put all ingredients and blend until smooth.
- ✓ Take out and serve

132) Banana Green Smoothie

Preparation Time: 5 minutes

Cooking Time:

Servings: 1

Nutrition: Calories 364, Total Fat 4.8g, Saturated Fat 2.6g, Cholesterol 15mg, Sodium 111mg, Total Carbohydrate 78g, Dietary Fiber 8g, Total Sugars 45.1g, Protein 9.6g, Vitamin D 1mcg, Calcium 257mg, Iron 1mg, Potassium 1241mg

Ingredients:

- 1 cup coconut water
- ¾ cup plant-based milk
- ¼ tsp vanilla extract
- 1 heaping cup loosely packed spinach
- 2-3 cups frozen bananas, sliced

Directions:

- ✓ Blend everything until smooth and serve.

133) Cinnamon Coffee Shake

Preparation Time: 5 minutes

Cooking Time:

Servings: 2

Nutrition: Calories 197, Total Fat 6.4g, Saturated Fat 0.6g, Cholesterol 0mg, Sodium 5mg, Total Carbohydrate 31.3g, Dietary Fiber 5.2g, Total Sugars 15.8g, Protein 4g, Vitamin D 0mcg, Calcium 53mg, Iron 1mg, Potassium 582mg

Ingredients:

- 1 cup cooled coffee, regular or decaf
- ¼ cup almond or non-dairy milk
- A few pinches cinnamon
- 2 tbsp hemp seeds
- Splash vanilla extract
- 2 frozen bananas, sliced into coins
- Handful of ice

Directions:

- ✓ Chill some coffee in a sealed container for a couple of hours (or overnightbefore making this smoothie, or be ready to use more ice.
- ✓ Add the non-dairy milk, cinnamon, vanilla, and hemp seeds to a blender and blend until smooth. Add the coffee and cut bananas and keep blending until smooth.
- ✓ Add the ice and keep blending on high until there are no lumps remaining. Taste for sweetness and add your preferred plant-based sugar or sugar alternative.
- ✓ Transfer to a glass and serve.

134) Orange Smoothie

Preparation Time: 5 minutes

Cooking Time:

Servings: 2

Nutrition: Calories 269, Total Fat 12.3g, Saturated Fat 2.3g, Cholesterol 0mg, Sodium 312mg, Total Carbohydrate 37.6g, Dietary Fiber 8.2g, Total Sugars 22.9g, Protein 6.4g, Vitamin D 0mcg, Calcium 52mg, Iron 3mg, Potassium 528mg

Ingredients:

- 1 cup orange slices
- 1 cup mango chunks
- 1 cup strawberries, chopped
- 1 cup coconut water
- Pinch freshly grated ginger
- 1-2 cups crushed ice

Directions:

- ✓ Place everything in a blender, blend, and serve.

135) Pumpkin Smoothie

Preparation Time: 5 minutes

Cooking Time:

Servings: 2

Nutrition: Calories 272, Total Fat 5.6g, Saturated Fat 2.2g, Cholesterol 10mg, Sodium 75mg, Total Carbohydrate 51.9g, Dietary Fiber 9.5g,Total Sugars 29.4g, Protein 8.2g, Vitamin D 1mcg, Calcium 204mg, Iron 4mg,Potassium 865mg

Ingredients:

- 1 cup unsweetened non-dairy milk
- 2 medium bananas, peeled and cut into quarters and frozen
- 2 medjool dates, pitted
- 1 cup pumpkin puree, canned or fresh
- 2 cups ice cubes
- ¼ tsp cinnamon
- 2 tbsp ground flaxseeds
- 1 tsp pumpkin spice

Directions:

- ✓ Blend all ingredients in a blender and serve.

136) Turmeric Smoothie

Preparation Time: 5 minutes

Cooking Time:

Servings: 2

Nutrition: Calories 785, Total Fat 62.4g, Saturated Fat 51.5g, Cholesterol 0mg, Sodium 41mg, Total Carbohydrate 60.2g, Dietary Fiber 15g, Total Sugars 33.9g, Protein 10g, Vitamin D 0mcg, Calcium 149mg, Iron 6mg,

Ingredients:

- 2 cups non-dairy milk like coconut, almond
- 2 medium bananas, frozen
- 1 cup mango, frozen
- 1 tsp turmeric, ground grated, peeled
- 1 tsp fresh ginger, grated, peeled
- 1 tbsp chia seeds
- ¼ tsp vanilla extract
- ¼ tsp cinnamon, ground
- 1 pinch pepper, ground

Directions:

- ✓ Blend all ingredients in a blender and serve

137) Veggie Smoothie

Preparation Time: 10 minutes

Cooking Time:

Servings: 1

Nutrition: Calories 696, Total Fat 34.1g, Saturated Fat 7g, Cholesterol 10mg, Sodium 190mg, Total Carbohydrate 90.5g, Dietary Fiber 29.5g, Total Sugars 37.2g, Protein 18.5g, Vitamin D 1mcg, Calcium 527mg, Iron 9mg, Potassium 2223mg

Ingredients:

- 1 stalk celery
- 1 carrot peeled and roughly chopped
- ½ cup broccoli sprouts
- 1 cup kale, chopped
- ½ cup curly parsley
- ½ tomato roughly chopped
- ½ avocado
- 1 banana
- ½ green apple
- ½ cup non-dairy milk
- 1 tbsp chia seeds
- 1 tbsp flaxseeds

Directions:

- ✓ Place all ingredients in a blender.
- ✓ Blend until smooth. Serve immediately.

138) Coco Loco Smoothie

Preparation Time: 5 minutes

Cooking Time:

Servings: 2

Nutrition: Carbs: 18.2 g Protein: 10.2 g Fats: 27.0 g Calories: 309 Kcal

Ingredients:

- Coconut milk: 1 cup
- Frozen cauliflower florets: ½ cup
- Frozen mango cubes: 1 cup
- Almond butter: 1 tbsp

Directions:

- ✓ Add all the ingredients to the blender
- ✓ Blend on high speed to make it smooth

139) Very Berry Smoothie

Preparation Time: 5 minutes

Cooking Time:

Servings: 2

Nutrition: Calories 269, Total Fat 12.3g, Saturated Fat 2.3g, Cholesterol 0mg, Sodium 312mg, Total Carbohydrate 37.6g, Dietary Fiber 8.2g, Total Sugars 22.9g, Protein 6.4g, Vitamin D 0mcg, Calcium 52mg, Iron 3mg, Potassium 528mg

Ingredients:

- 2 cups, plant-based Milk
- 2 cups, Frozen or fresh berries
- ½ cup Frozen ripe bananas
- 2 teaspoons, Flax Seeds
- ¼ tsp, Vanilla
- ¼ tsp, Cinnamon

Directions:

- ✓ Mix together milk, flax seeds, and fruit. Blend in a high-power blender.
- ✓ Add cinnamon and vanilla. Blend until smooth.
- ✓ Serve and enjoy!

140) Creamy Carrot Smoothie

Preparation Time: 5 minutes

Cooking Time:

Servings: 4

Nutrition: Carbs: 14.9 g Protein: 3 g Fats: 4.5 g Calories: 103 Kcal

Ingredients:

- Almond milk: 2 cups
- Prunes: 60 g
- Banana: 1
- Carrots: 150 g
- Walnuts: 30 g
- Ground cinnamon:½ tsp
- Vanilla extract:1 tsp

Directions:

- ✓ Add all the ingredients to the blender
- ✓ Blend on high speed to make it smooth

141) Date Chocolate Smoothie

Preparation Time: 5 minutes

Cooking Time:

Servings: 2

Nutrition: Carbs: 72.1 g Protein: 8 g Fats: 12.7 g Calories: 385 Kcal

Ingredients:

- Unsweetened cocoa powder: 2 tbsp
- Unsweetened nut milk: 2 cups
- Almond butter: 2 tbsp
- Dried dates: 4 pitted
- Frozen bananas: 2 medium
- Ground cinnamon: ¼ tsp

Directions:

- ✓ Add all the ingredients to the blender
- ✓ Blend to form a smooth consistency

142) Date Banana Pistachio Smoothie

Preparation Time: 5 minutes

Cooking Time:

Servings: 4

Nutrition: Carbs: 32.9 g Protein: 9.7 g Fats: 15 g Calories: 320 Kcal

Ingredients:

- Pistachios: 1 cup
- Raw pumpkin:175 g
- Cloves:1
- Nutmeg:1/8 tsp
- Dates: 4
- Banana:1
- Ground ginger:1/8 tsp
- Ground cinnamon:1 tsp
- Cashew milk:500 ml
- Ice: as per your need

Directions:

- ✓ Add all the ingredients to the blender
- ✓ Blend on high speed to make it smooth

143) Fall Green Smoothie

Preparation Time: 5 minutes

Cooking Time:

Servings: 1

Nutrition: Carbs: 37.1 g Protein: 6.5 g Fats: 5.4 g Calories: 183 Kcal

Ingredients:

- Persimmon: 1
- Spinach: 1 cup
- Orange: 1
- Water: 1 cup
- Chia seeds:1 tbsp

Directions:

- ✓ Add all the ingredients to the blender
- ✓ Blend to form a smooth consistency
- ✓ Add ice cubes from the top to chill it

144) Fig Protein Smoothie

Preparation Time: 5 minutes

Cooking Time:

Servings: 1

Nutrition: Carbs: 66.0 g Protein: 16.1 g Fats: 18 g Calories: 435 Kcal

Ingredients:

- Fresh figs: 2
- Almond milk: 1 cup
- Dried date: 1 pitted
- Vanilla extract: ¼ tsp
- Sesame seeds: 2 tbsp

Directions:

- ✓ Add all the ingredients to the blender
- ✓ Blend to form a smooth consistency

145) Frozen Berries Smoothie

Preparation Time: 5 minutes

Cooking Time:

Servings: 2

Nutrition: Carbs: 14.9 g Protein: 2.2 g Fats: 1.6 g Calories: 92 Kcal

Ingredients:

- Banana: 1 ripe
- Frozen berries: 200g
- Almond milk: 250ml

Directions:

- ✓ Add all the ingredients in the blender
- ✓ Blend to give a smooth consistency
- ✓ Pour to the glasses and serve

146) Fruit Medley Smoothie

Preparation Time: 5 minutes

Cooking Time:

Servings: 2

Nutrition: Carbs: 52.8 g Protein: 6.4 g Fats: 22.5 g Calories: 407 Kcal

Ingredients:

- Banana: 1 ripe sliced
- Almond milk: 1 cup
- Coconut oil: 1 tbsp
- Powdered ginger: 1 tsp
- Frozen fruit medley: 1 cup
- Chia seeds: 2 tbsp

Directions:

- ✓ Add all the ingredients in the blender
- ✓ Blend to give a smooth consistency
- ✓ Pour to the glasses and serve

147) Green Healthy Smoothie

Preparation Time: 5 minutes

Cooking Time:

Servings: 1

Nutrition: Carbs: 41.2 g Protein: 8.9 g Fats: 3.9 g Calories: 220 Kcal

Ingredients:

- Large banana: 1 frozen
- Fresh spinach: 1 cup
- Rolled oats: 2 tbsp
- Unsweetened almond milk: ¾ cup

Directions:

- ✓ Add all the ingredients to the blender
- ✓ Blend to form a smooth consistency

148) Halva Smoothie

Preparation Time: 5 minutes

Cooking Time:

Servings: 1

Nutrition: Carbs: 66.0 g

Protein: 12.1 g Fats: 16.5g Calories: 435 Kcal

Ingredients:

- Dried date: 1 pitted
- Tahini: 1 tbsp
- Fresh figs: 2
- Almond milk: 1 cup
- Vanilla extract: ¼ tsp

Directions:

- ✓ Add all the ingredients to the blender
- ✓ Blend to form a smooth consistency

149) Kale Smoothie

Preparation Time: 5 minutes

Cooking Time:

Servings: 1

Nutrition: Carbs: 34.1 Protein: 12.8 g Fats: 14 g Calories: 244 Kcal

Ingredients:

- Almond butter: 1 tbsp
- Large banana: 1 frozen
- Fresh kale: 1 cup
- Unsweetened almond milk: ¾ cup

Directions:

- ✓ Add all the ingredients to the blender
- ✓ Blend to form a smooth consistency

150) Kiwi And Almonds Smoothie

Preparation Time: 5 minutes

Cooking Time:

Servings: 2

Nutrition: Carbs: 37.1 g Protein: 15.2 g Fats: 28.3 g Calories: 427 Kcal

Ingredients:

- Almonds: ½ cup
- Coconut milk: 1 cup
- Kiwi: 1 medium peeled and sliced
- Banana:1 sliced
- Ice cubes: 4
- Avocado: 1/2 small
- Baby spinach:1 cup lightly packed

Directions:

- ✓ Add all the ingredients to the blender
- ✓ Blend to form a smooth consistency

8. Dr. Carlisle's Smash Meal Plan – Men Version

The meal plan is divided into 7 days, to be repeated for 3 weeks, with 5 meals a day.

Following this plan does not guarantee extreme results.

The aim is to keep metabolism under control in order to change eating habits, have more energy available during the day, and keep under control the values that lead to hormonal sudden changes.

The plan here below is an example of food plan that can be followed by a healthy person without specific pathologies. I do not take responsibility for personal injury, before following the plan consult your doctor

Instructions for use

Follow the plan daily: drink plenty of water at every meal, it is imperative not to take alcohol (it's not good for the body!)

It is possible to substitute meals at will according to this book, so that it does not become habitual to always eat the same things.

Day 1

1) Oatmeal & Peanut Butter Breakfast Bar | Calories 459

102) Tofu Fajita Bowl | Calories 263

54) Loaded Kale Salad | Calories 72

28) Creamy Tofu Mushroom Soup | Calories 923

130) Raspberry Lime Smoothie | Calories 227

Total calories: 1944

Day 2

4) Cinnamon Rolls with Cashew | Calories 226

106) Seitan Meatza With Kale | Calories 601

59) Broccoli Sweet Potato Chickpea Salad | Calories 231

36) Greek Lentil Soup | Calories 231

137) Veggie Smoothie | Calories 696

Total calories: 1985

Day 3

9) Fluffy Garbanzo Bean Omelet | Calories 104

115) Lunch Recipes |Calories 232

65) Vegetable Salad With Chimichurri | Calories 231

31) Chilled Lemongrass And Avocado Soup |Calories 339

146) Fruit Medley Smoothie | Calories 407

Total calories: 1313

Day 4

14) Pineapple and Kale Smoothie | Calories 509

118) Lentils Bolognese With Soba Noodles | Calories 353

74) Roasted Asparagus w. Feta Cheese Salad | Calories 146

42) Beanless Garden Soup |Calories 305

150) Kiwi And Almonds Smoothie | Calories 427

Total calories: 1740

Day 5

18) Greens and Berry Smoothie |Calories 298

121) Tempeh Skewers With Dressing | Calories 351

80) Simple Peas Mix | Calories 133

50) 3-Ingredient Carrot And Red Lentil Soup | Calories 90

133) Cinnamon Coffee Shake | Calories 197

Total calories:1069

Day 6

22) Spinach Tofu Scramble With Sour Cream | Calories 411

116) Lemon Pepper Pasta | Calories 489

86) Roasted Broccoli With Peanuts And Kecap Manis | Calories 258

44) Spinach Soup With Basil | Calories 162

127) Amazing Blueberry Smoothie | Calories 269

Total calories: 1589

Day 7

25) Amaranth Quinoa Porridge | Calories 474

104) Ginger Lime Tempeh | Calories 285

90) Rocket Chickpeas Salad | Calories 586

40) Chinese Rice Soup | Calories 210

142) Date Banana Pistachio Smoothie | Calories 320

Total calories: 1875

9. Conclusion

I hope you enjoyed this book....

The world of plant-based nutrition is diverse, I hope I have brought you at least a little closer to your goals.

Whether you want to lose weight, adopt a healthy lifestyle, or simply break your physiological routine, I'm happy if I've been able to contribute even a little to your life change.

Always remember:

Follow your doctor's instructions: with his guidance, you will learn how to easily get out of the way even when you are unmotivated to continue success.

Always have these skills on your side:

Perseverance....

Patience.....

Good luck with your projects .... I will be here when you need me!

CPSIA information can be obtained
at www.ICGtesting.com
Printed in the USA
LVHW062302020521
686271LV00015B/719

9 781802 663129